RESI
THE ROLLER CC

This enthralling narrative is a superb reminder that the human spirit has the extraordinary capacity to convert adversity into strength.

J.T., Cancer Survivor

This book is a powerful, uplifting story about taking charge of the battle with attitude and information.

C.J., Cancer Survivor

I couldn't put this book down until I was finished. I found myself laughing and crying, and learning that kooky occurrences, intense emotions, odd interactions with people you love, and confusion are all normal. Normal, that is, during a major illness. This book will be a great help for patients and their families.

M.F., Cancer Survivor

Not a single story, but many, artfully woven into a beautiful and compelling portrait of struggle and triumph.

L.S., Cancer Survivor

I identified with so many of the emotions and the scenarios in this book, and it gave me the hope that my own roller coaster ride would come to an end.

A.M., Cancer Survivor

This book is a road map for anyone who wants to understand how a cancer patient feels.

J.P., Cancer Survivor and Caregiver

The author's frank discussions of her husband's support in
the face of his own loneliness make this book a must read
for all men who love women facing cancer.

J.H., Caregiver

The author confronts cancer with determination, courage
and wit. Her humor adds a special dimension to a horrible
experience.

D.C., Cancer Survivor

I was unable to put this book down, and read it in a single
sitting. It is aptly named because you will shift rapidly from
laughing til you hurt to choking back tears. This book is
truly a gift for anyone facing a major illness.

T.A., Cancer Survivor

Aided by her supportive husband, superb medical care, and
the sheer determination to live, this feisty author reveals inti-
mate glimpses into struggling with mortality and emerging
whole from the struggle.

J.C., Cancer Survivor

This book teaches you not to take yourself too seriously, a
very important lesson in the face of any adversity.

L.F., Cancer Survivor

The Roller Coaster Chronicles

Betsy de Parry

To Nadine — With healing hugs! Betsy

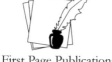

First Page Publications

First Page Publications
12103 Merriman • Livonia • MI • 48150
1-800-343-3034 • Fax 734-525-4420
www.firstpagepublications.com

Cover designed by Kimberly Franzen

Cover image:
The author's surgical specimen,
also known as "The Pea,"
as described on page 25.

Photo courtesy of:
Robert E. Ruiz, M.D., Ph.D.
Clinical Assistant Professor
Department of Pathology
University of Michigan

Library of Congress Control Number: 2004117392
    de Parry, Betsy, 1950 -
        The Roller Coaster Chronicles / Betsy de Parry
    ISBN 1-928623-24-7
    Summary: The personal narrative of a woman who survives
lymphoma.

THIS BOOK IS DEDICATED TO:

My husband Alex,
the world's greatest cheerleader and the wind beneath
my wings

My daughter and grandchildren, Juli, Skye and Nicholas
Perrotto, for their immunity-enhancing love and joy

My mother Elizabeth Kurka,
Lady Wisdom, Lady Long Genes

My sister Karen Dickenson,
for knowing me and loving me anyway

My best friend Noreen Djokic,
my personal Ya-Ya sister

Dr. Mark Kaminski and Judy Estes,
for helping me to heal in ways that no medicine
ever could

TABLE OF CONTENTS

Foreword — Welcome Aboard ix

Chapter 1 — Cancer Calls 1

Chapter 2 — The Great Excavation 19

Chapter 3 — The Queen of Denial 29

Chapter 4 — Big Girls Do Cry 45

Chapter 5 — Rocky 65

Chapter 6 — Dope-On-A-Rope 81

Chapter 7 — Hotel Hell .93

Chapter 8 — From Miserable to Mangy 115

Chapter 9 — The Summer of Oblivion 131

Chapter 10 — The Invisible Invader
Scores Again 149

Chapter 11 — Believe in Miracles 169

Chapter 12 — Letting Go and Going On 187

Epilogue — The Honorable Discharge 211

Afterword — Information, Support
and Advocacy 233

Acknowledgements 235

About the Author 242

WELCOME ABOARD

December 20, 2001. I dialed Alex's cell phone. "Where are you?" I begged to know, not caring where he was, but that he wasn't where I thought he ought to be. "We should be leaving the house in twenty-five minutes and you haven't even packed."

"Don't worry," he calmly replied.

Exasperated, I chided him with the same remark I frequently made when he was late. "Alex, you're gonna be late for your own funeral."

Jokingly, he always answered, "Yeah, but you're gonna be early for yours."

My suitcases were already in the car and I was pacing the floor when Alex strolled unhurriedly through the back door. "I'm on vacation," he announced, grinning from ear to ear.

"Just go pack—and hurry," I urged him, nervously tapping my fingers on the counter.

"Quit worrying," he said breezily as he kissed my cheek and sauntered upstairs as if the plane would wait for him. "You're with me, and I've never missed a plane yet." True, but we'd been the last passengers to board on more than one occasion. Alex called it good time management. I called it nerve-wracking.

We did make it to the airport on time. Barely. And with Alex, I stepped on that plane and buckled up myself and my multiple roles—wife, mother, grandmother, vice president of marketing and sales, volunteer—to name a few. We landed in West Palm Beach late that night, happy to take a break from work and the cold Michigan winter. When we boarded the plane to return home several days later, we had no idea that the fever brewing in me was about to add another role to my life: cancer patient.

Cancer plunged us headlong into unfamiliar territory without a compass or a map, much less the time to get our bearings. It cast us into a macabre world of language we often didn't understand, forced us to make choices without fully understanding their consequences, and compelled us to trust my life to total strangers. It hurled us onto a roller coaster where denial, anger, guilt, and fear at times propelled us downward at speeds that made us wonder if anything would break our fall. At other times, humor and hope inched us upward.

In the beginning, Alex and I had no idea that we were riding such chaotic rails. Instead, we were certain that we would easily glide over whatever bumps lay ahead. I was so certain, in fact, that I declared I would write a motivational book full of wit and wisdom. We'd faced adversity before, and cancer was just another speed bump in the road of life. We couldn't have been more wrong. Nothing prepared us for the betrayal we felt when my own body tried to kill me.

It didn't take long for me to abandon the motivational idea, but I did keep a journal. Eight months after diagnosis, I read it, in its entirety, in the middle of a sleepless night, and I realized that recording events had helped me to interpret the emotions that had so often colored—and warped—my perspective. I began to wonder if sharing our story might help those who would follow in our footsteps. Yet I also realized that our story was just that—ours and ours alone. The circumstances in our lives were different from anyone else's. My cancer, its treatments, and its side effects were also unique. Even people who underwent the very same chemotherapy had different side effects, some better, some worse. I also wondered if anyone would read our story. After all, Alex and I weren't celebrities, but just ordinary people going about our ordinary lives when cancer assaulted us.

At last, I concluded that while each illness is unique and each person has his or her own way of coping with life, our story might help others as they design their own patterns for living with disease. Many months later, I would hope that others might find strength in my recovery and hope that healing is possible.

But at that time, in August 2002, when I was most ill, I began to rewrite my journal for reasons that were far less clear. The first ten chapters are the result. The final two chapters were written as they happened. I completed the manuscript exactly one year after I learned I had cancer. It then resided on my computer for over a year before I wrote the epilogue.

Far from the oh-this-is-easy-you-can-do-it book I initially envisioned, this book is a collage of reflections and incidents during our year on the roller coaster. You'll see that it took some time for Mr. Tardiness and Mrs. Punctuality to ride in the same car. You'll ride with us as we were jolted by shock, shaken by worry and fear, went numb, hurt, laughed and cried, tried to pretend life was normal, felt sorry for ourselves, fought and made up—and white-knuckled, held on to the roller coaster for dear life, determined to reach the finish line in one piece. You'll glimpse our problems and solutions, our joys and sorrows, our hopes and frustrations as we grappled with uncertainty, reeled from unexpected blows, and pushed doggedly ahead, stabilized by the expertise and compassion of the health care professionals who cared for me and by the friends and family who supported us.

Any life-threatening disease is indeed a formidable foe, and it requires that you surround yourself with health care professionals whose knowledge, experience, and judgment you trust, and in whose understanding and encouragement, coupled with appropriate realism, you find confidence and support. I have spared no words of praise for most of those who cared for me—because they deserve it and because they are shining examples of what every person deserves during any type of illness. A couple of others nearly pushed Alex and me into emotional freefall without a safety net.

You and your loved ones will ride your own rails, and each of you will do it in your own way. Everyone approaches illness differently, based on life experiences up to the point of diagnosis, present circumstances, personality, and a variety of other factors. There is no right or wrong way to cope with the stresses of life-threatening disease, but there are ways to smooth out the ride, however slightly.

Whether you are a patient, caregiver, spouse, friend or health care professional, Alex and I share our story with you, complete with our occasional erratic behavior, with the hope that the insight will be helpful to you in whatever capacity illness touches your life. For patients and partners especially, we hope with all our hearts that you will find some comfort and guidance herein to help you build your own survival techniques so that you may truly *live* in spite of illness.

CHAPTER ONE

CANCER CALLS

My cell phone rang while I was driving north on 23.
It was Emergency's Dr. Ketcham asking,
"Do you remember me?"
"Of course," I answered. "And how are you?"
"Fine," he said, "but there's bad news for you.
Your test results show misshapen cells.
Your white blood counts are high.
Lymphoma is the suspect. Further tests will verify.
Do you know what lymphoma is?" he asked,
and I quietly blurted out,
"Yes, it's a form of cancer that I could do without."
I remember nothing more about our conversation.
I pulled off on the shoulder, trembling with fear
and trepidation.
For some time I sat in stupor,
then I heard trucks whizzing by,
And realized it was a dangerous place for the
"Oh-my-God-I-have-cancer" cry.
And so I slowly pulled back on the interstate.
I headed home to ponder this newly handed fate.

No, this would not be my fate, thought I.
It was just the hospital's precaution
Against this world gone mad with lawsuits,
litigation, and extortion.
I'd play along.
I'd have their tests,
but there's nothing wrong with me,
For I'm a mere girl at fifty-one, strong and invincible—
they'll see!

Alexander Graham Bell must have been a swell guy. Thanks to him, I joyously learned I would be a grandmother once, then twice, moments after conception, or at least as soon as my daughter was certain her babies were on their way. His invention had been the transmitter of shared secrets and dreams, gossip and recipes. On it, I spoke to clients and prospective clients, scheduled appointments, whispered sweet nothings to my husband, laughed with my sister and my best friend. Mr. Bell's phone was a great gift, I thought, until the morning of January 7, 2002. On that day, I would have preferred Pony Express. It might have ensured me a few more days of blissful tranquility.

It was just before ten that morning when Dr. Eric Ketcham, a third-year resident in the emergency room, called to inform me that tests indicated cancer. There I was, driving on US-23 north of Ann Arbor, Michigan, slightly south of the Silver Lake exit. I'll never pass that exact spot again without thinking about the phone call that turned my world inside out and upside down.

Dr. Ketcham first asked if I was at a place we could talk. Of course, I told him, failing to mention that I was behind the wheel on a busy highway. He presented the facts respectfully and calmly. My white blood counts were high. He suspected lymphoma. I should see a specialist right away. We were still talking when I pulled off onto the shoulder, thinking that he might as well have said, "Good morning, Mrs. de Parry. I'm calling to bring you a message of terror. And if you think cancer is hard on your body, just wait until you see what it does to your psyche. I suggest you and your family equip yourselves with emotional yo-yos with l-o-n-g elastic strings. You'll need them." Of course, no doctor would ever be so blunt. At least I hope not.

I'm not certain how long I sat there after Dr. Ketcham and I hung up. It couldn't have been more than a few minutes. I didn't cry. I just sat, oblivious to everything around me. What does one do, I wondered, when a total stranger announces that cancer has called upon you? Curiously, I wondered how doctors psych themselves up to make those calls. Finally, I decided to call my husband Alex. He always had answers for everything, but then, all he could think of was, "Stay there. I'll come get you."

"That doesn't make sense," I replied. "We'd have to come back to get my car." I assured him I was fine to drive. Doesn't every car come equipped with autopilot for just such predicaments? My car made a U-turn and navigated itself home, carrying me and my fear that an invisible invader had just hijacked me.

Alex wanted to do *something*. But what? Work the phone!

Trying to determine what we should do next, he began calling the doctors we knew at the University of Michigan (U of M) until he reached one of them. Before I had arrived home, he had contacted a doctor friend who knew exactly what to do. There was a clinic that specialized in lymphoma, and our friend would call to see about getting us in right away.

I pulled into the garage and walked into the kitchen to wait for Alex. Everything was just as I had left it, but the house looked different. Felt different. I felt detached from everything that was familiar. I wandered from room to room, scanning all the family photographs scattered about. I desperately wanted to feel connected to the people in those photographs, for they were part of the past, the present, and the future. But I felt suspended in time, severed from the orderly transition of life. Don't be a drama queen, I thought. This is just a bad dream.

Surely nothing so horrible as cancer would sabotage our lives now. We'd both endured various challenges in our lives, but at the moment, life was good. No, it was great. Alex and I had known each other a dozen years, lived together for six and a half, and been married for just over three. Thirty-one years earlier, he'd started a home building company. I had sold homes all my adult life in West Palm Beach, Florida. Smitten, I'd traded my sandals for boots and joined him in Ann Arbor, where I went to work with him.

Wandering through the house, I thought about how great our lives had been until that phone call less than an hour earlier. We'd just completed a successful year, were financially stable, enjoyed a blissful marriage, and had plenty of optimism and energy for a couple of fifty-somethings. Who could ask for more?

I became angry. Angry that anything would dare to intrude on our busy, happy lives. Angry that my plans for the morning had changed. I had things to do, people to see, places to go. It was a new year, and I had plenty of goals to accomplish. We were to begin Mystic Ridge, the largest development we had ever undertaken, later in the year. I had no time for medical tests, much less a major illness. Cancer was definitely *not* a part of my new year's resolution.

But of course I was not ill. It was not possible. In this litigious age, surely the doctors had to be overly cautious, even if I promised never to sue them. I would never expend the necessary time or energy to do so, but they didn't know that. Ambulance chasers were causing all this, and why was I letting one stupid little phone call interrupt my plans anyway?

Alex arrived home, put his arms around me, and assured me he was as certain as I that this was just a mistake. Nevertheless, someone from the Lymphoma Clinic would look at the tests and call us late in the afternoon. There was nothing more to do but wait. Exhausted, I settled onto the couch as the fever started brewing again.

That's what had started it all. In West Palm Beach during the afternoon of December 30, I had felt very tired while shopping with my daughter Juli and her children, two-and-a-half-year-old Skye and ten-month-old Nicholas. By the time Juli dropped me off at our condo, I was running a low-grade fever, which I assumed to be caused by a little bug I picked up from the kids.

By morning the fever had broken, but it returned that afternoon. I didn't let it stop us from spending New Year's Eve at Noreen and Walter's house. Noreen, my dearest friend and my real estate partner when I lived in West Palm Beach, can turn any evening into side-splitting comedy. Laughing until tears rolled down our cheeks, we bored Alex and Walter with our old stories and shared some new ones. We were home by ten, and I fell asleep way before the ball dropped. Some party animal, huh?

Each afternoon the fever returned. My thighs ached. I jokingly accused Noreen of trying to poison me with her cooking on New Year's Eve. Alex was certain I had some type of flu or maybe a virus, and he bought every cold and flu tonic that lined the drugstore shelf. But nothing worked. A little voice inside me said this wasn't the flu. It started whispering, "Better check this out." If I had tried to explain the little voice, Alex would have thought I had lost my mind.

When we flew home on January 3, I had a low fever and could barely walk through the airport. With each step, my legs wanted to give out, and I could scarcely stay awake. At baggage claim, all the chairs were occupied, so I collapsed on the floor while Alex retrieved the luggage.

I knew I needed medical help, but I had no regular doctor, since I was not one to haul myself in for regular inspections. The morning after we arrived home, I phoned a family practice group for an appointment. They could see me in March. "And just what shall I do if the fevers continue?"

I asked. "Go to the emergency room," a cold voice answered.

At noon that day I had scheduled a meeting with prospective clients who had called about one of our "spec" homes. We met at our home, which we often used as an example of our work. Translated, I had to keep our house in perfect shape every day, never knowing just who might appear. Molly Maid was another hat I wore.

During the meeting, I could feel the fever returning. It had returned early every afternoon for days. Why should that day have been any different? For three hours, I answered questions. For the last two hours, I wished they'd go away and let me retreat to the couch.

By the time they left, my temperature had hit 103. Unable to reach Alex, I headed to U of M's emergency room, a fifteen-minute drive from home. Yes, Independent is my middle name, or at least I would like to think it is. Alex and I finally connected as I neared the hospital. "U of M is a trauma center. You'll spend all night there," he said. Still certain I had some kind of weird flu or virus, he recommended I go to the corner emergency clinic.

I was aggravated that he would even suggest the corner clinic. There was that little voice inside my head, now screaming, "You need to be at U of M! Don't go anywhere else, fool." Alex joined me at the emergency room, annoyed that I had shown up at a trauma center on a Friday night for a little fever.

I spent the next twelve hours in the emergency room. About halfway through the summary of potential suspects for this unexplained malady, Dr. Ketcham casually said something about cancer, but assured me that was very unlikely. For definitive answers, we'd have to wait for test results. I returned home, certain that nothing was really wrong that couldn't easily be fixed. Otherwise Dr. Ketcham would have admitted me to the hospital. Right? That weekend would be the last of such ignorant bliss.

Though exhausted, I was at least fever-free in the mornings, and I wasn't about to let a little fatigue stop me from doing what I felt was necessary. That's when I got in my car on Monday morning to make the forty-five-minute drive to our tile supplier to find bathroom flooring for a "spec" home. And that's when the world as I knew it changed forever, thanks to the phone call from Dr. Ketcham.

As I waited to hear from someone at the Lymphoma Clinic later that day, I frantically tried to convince myself that cancer was impossible. No one in my family had ever had it. Strokes were the culprit in our genes, not cancer. By early afternoon, the fever had returned, and I collapsed on the couch, from which I ranted, raved, and yelled at Alex. "I will NOT have this." That day would be the first of many that he would be my lightning rod, attempting to ground me against my own highly charged emotions. It wasn't long before he simply could absorb no more voltage.

The phone finally rang late in the afternoon. A calm, kind, compassionate voice told me that she had looked at the blood tests taken at the emergency room and felt that a more specialized test—flow cytometry—would be necessary to determine whether the suspicion of lymphoma was accurate. Good, here is a loophole, I thought. Whatever flow cytometry was, it would prove the initial suspicions wrong. Very wrong. I agreed to have the test the following day.

That calm voice belonged to Judy Estes, nurse practitioner and Lymphoma Program coordinator. The clinic specializes in the diagnosis and treatment of all the various kinds of blood cancers. Using a team approach, each case is reviewed by a group of highly trained specialists, including hematologists/oncologists, radiation oncologists, surgical oncologists, pathologists, nurse practitioners, physician's assistants, and oncology nurses. Together, like five-star generals convening in a war room, they evaluate each patient's individual case and develop a carefully coordinated treatment plan.

At the time, I had no way of knowing that so much brainpower would eventually evaluate my case. I knew only that I would gladly undergo another poke in the arm to withdraw blood for this flow cytometry test. Little did I know the truth it would tell. By week's end, the fevers had stopped, and I grew confident that nothing was wrong. That's when Judy called with the news that the flow cytometry test had confirmed earlier suspicions. She had already made an appointment for me to see Dr. Mark Kaminski the following week.

That second "you have cancer" call, five days after the first, immediately dashed my growing confidence. I hung up the phone, put my elbows on the kitchen counter, and buried my head in my hands. This can't be happening, I thought. My test must have been switched with someone else's. Or someone misread the results. I *can't* have cancer.

Then why did I feel so scared?

After several minutes, I hauled myself upstairs to dress for the Home Builder Association's annual awards banquet that evening. I stepped into the shower, and for a very long time, stood motionless under the running water. My whole naked body felt heavy and weighted, and my mind was empty, save for one thought: I can't have cancer.

I couldn't have heard Alex arrive home, and I didn't hear him come into the bathroom until he was knocking on the shower door. "Hey, you gonna save me any hot water?" he asked.

I just stood there, looking at him through the glass. I could tell by his face that he knew something was wrong. I turned off the water, wrapped a towel around me, stepped out of the shower, and sat down on the edge of the whirlpool. "What is it?" Alex asked.

I stared at the floor, unable to answer him. I tried, but I could only begin sentences, not complete them. He got the message and reminded me that we hadn't yet seen the doctor. Test results could be wrong. There were surely more tests that would disprove that flow-whatever-it-was. And if I wanted to stay home that evening, it would be fine with him.

No, we would go out. I thought it would help to get our minds off the news, but my own despondence drowned out the laughter and lively conversation that filled the room that night. I hardly heard a thing anyone said. Alex even had to nudge me when my name was called for an award. Where had my spunk gone?

The following morning, some of it had returned. No way would I have cancer. Somebody's wrong. I just have to prove it. After breakfast, I went into my office to organize papers that had piled up, but it was clear that I would have to make room for them. I decided to clean out the bottom drawer of my file cabinet, which was bursting at the seams with an accumulation of papers that had no particular significance. Everything in the drawer was related to real estate or construction—ads I had once liked, copies of real estate contracts from other areas of the country, and other papers I had saved, thinking that they might be useful someday. I threw many of them away to make room for more papers I would probably never need.

I lifted the very last file, wedged at the back of the drawer. Across the top I had written "Jokes and Miscellaneous." I laughed at some of the jokes I hadn't seen in years. And then I came to the very last piece of paper in that file, a copy of an article on thermal fax paper, faint but still legible. I think my heart almost stopped. I know I got a cold chill. And I shrieked so loudly that Alex ran upstairs to see what was going on. In bold letters, the title of the article proclaimed, "Curing Cancer," and it was about a new breakthrough pioneered by none other than Mark Kaminski.

I had completely forgotten about this article, but I did remember how it came into my possession. In the fall of 1996, Alex and I were working in a Detroit suburb. One of our colleagues had a friend who was diagnosed with lymphoma. I'm sure that was the first I had ever heard of the disease. She had heard of an article written about a cancer breakthrough at U of M and thought that it had been printed in the *Observer*, a monthly magazine about Ann Arbor. She wondered if we had seen it. No, we hadn't, but it was worth a phone call to the *Observer*. Yes, there was an article about a cancer breakthrough, and someone at the *Observer* faxed it right over. I made a photocopy for our colleague and hoped that the information would help her friend. Only now did I realize that I had kept the copy the *Observer* had faxed over.

But why? I never, ever kept articles that were not pertinent to our business or our interests. Cancer obviously has absolutely nothing to do with the home building industry, and I assure you it does not fall under the category of hobbies and interests. Keeping that article was one thousand percent out of character for me. Don't try to convince me there isn't a higher being.

Five and a half years after pulling that article off the fax machine, I read it. But first I stared at the faded picture of Dr. Kaminski, glad to know at least what he looked like. I scrutinized him as if he could soon be my savior. He had developed a new drug called Bexxar which treated lymphoma using a radiolabeled antibody. I didn't completely understand the concept, but I did grasp its success. Cure, the article said, was possible with this new treatment. Surely, five and a half years after its printing and several clinical trials later, this new drug would get rid of lymphoma—*if*, of course, I even had it.

Alex and I read and re-read the article. This Dr. Kaminski was a whole lot smarter and more dedicated than I would ever be. Shame on me for filing him under "Jokes and Miscellaneous." He deserved better. I wanted to toss out the article along with all the other papers I was discarding, but I just couldn't. Something made me place it in its own notebook, as if to confer respect to this man who had spent most of his life helping an unfortunate group of people— to which, of course, I could not, would not, belong.

Closing the file cabinet, I grew angry. Angry that a blood test was interfering with my busy schedule. Fear soon followed—fear of what I was certain was an overworked, understaffed health care system where profit took precedent over people. I was sure I would be reduced to a patient number and a statistic, just one of thousands of people who pass through the revolving doors hoping to be made good as new. If—and it was a big *if*—there were something wrong with me, would anybody care that I have a name and a life that matters, at least to me?

Physically, the University of Michigan Health Care System is a huge complex of massive buildings. And I mean massive, as in 4,671,878 square feet massive. For all you sports fans, that's equivalent to almost 58 football fields or nearly 649 tennis courts. In my world, it equates to about 107 acres, or 1,868 twenty-five-hundred-square-foot homes. And I was supposed to navigate around the place? Right.

I'd entered the hospital only once, a few years earlier when my mother came down with pneumonia while she was visiting us. The first time my sister and I went to see her after she was admitted from the emergency room, we got thoroughly lost in those vast buildings. Down corridor after corridor, through door after door, we wandered through the labyrinth and straight into the bowels of that grand institution.

Behind the last door we opened was a lab. And not just any lab. This one was filled with monkeys…*caged*. Astounded, my sister and I looked at them, looked at each other, closed the door, and, without a word, ran. And I mean *ran*. Some distance down the hall, we stopped, hardly believing what we had just seen.

"I want to rescue every one of those poor animals. Do you think we can get them out of here without being noticed?" I pondered. We both knew the answer. "Mother's not *here*, and this place gives me the creeps," I said.

Poor animals. I could hardly think about what must happen to them. From that day forward, when I drove past the hospital, I envisioned the monkeys and shuddered. The hospital represented one big research project, and now I might become just another one of its monkeys. Surely no one would see me as a human being with a real family and real feelings. What would I matter to anyone so long as I made a contribution to research? Obviously it had not occurred to me that research was what prolonged life.

Yes, I was a little defensive by the time our appointment came. Alex drove to that part of the hospital complex where a big sign directed us to the Cancer and Geriatrics Center. The sign might as well have said, "Mrs. de Parry, you'll have to graduate from cancer before you get to geriatrics." I tried to make jokes about being an antique, but Alex wasn't amused. Silently, I wondered how many strangers would have to see me naked. I had neither aspired to become a middle-aged Gypsy Rose Lee, nor did I want to submit to degrading and disgusting procedures.

The waiting area seemed like a holding pen for a variety of people of all ages, from children to seniors, who were at various stages of disease and treatment. Some were in wheelchairs. Some wore scarves, hats, various bandages, and surgical masks. Most looked tired and resigned. What horrors were happening to those poor souls, I wondered. I couldn't possibly belong in their midst.

And just what were Alex and I doing in a cancer clinic, anyway? We'd always been so healthy. Yet there sat our physical selves, together with our personalities, our beliefs, our fears, and our expectations, although Alex wasn't certain what to expect. At least I had experienced waiting rooms and doctors and hospitals during my parents' illnesses, but for Alex, the waiting room was completely foreign because he had never confronted so much illness in one place. Many months later, he would tell me that the magnitude of human suffering stared at him from the faces of the patients in that room. Of course he knew that illness existed, but for the first time, he came face to face with evidence of the physical and emotional effects that strike the vibrant lives of mothers, fathers, and children whose own lives had hardly begun. And in that waiting room, the toll of human illness became a terrible and frightening reality for him. He wondered why anyone is dealt such an awful hand.

We were taken to a small examining room where I admitted, "I'd rather be anywhere than here. This can't be happening."

"That's exactly what I was thinking," Alex replied, fidgeting with his wedding ring.

Judy arrived and examined me. She was a pretty woman with short hair, large eyes that communicated compassion, and an energetic and professional manner. She was as warm and kind in person as she had been on the phone, and I liked her instantly. Still, I was sure that Dr. Kaminski would bolt through the door, ask a question or two without ever looking at me, and leave as quickly as he had come. Isn't that what doctors do?

Nothing could have been further from the truth. Dr. Kaminski strode into the room wearing a friendly smile and genteel manner. He sat down, looked us squarely in the eye, and with his calm and steady voice, began to talk about lymphoma. Intuitively knowing that we had no idea what questions to ask, he answered all the ones he knew we would need answers to. In fact, he gave us more information than I could possibly absorb. Much to my amazement, he never seemed to be in any particular hurry. He didn't treat me like a monkey. And his gentle eyes and patient explanations, delivered unhurriedly with reassuring authority and compassion, almost persuaded me that he had aced his Bedside Manner course back in medical school.

Still, I wasn't convinced that he fully grasped how important life was to me. Maybe he was just having a good day. I knew only that if I really had a problem, I would need a doctor who would believe with all his heart that I would live, a doctor whom I could trust, with whom I could communicate, and who would deliver good news or bad compassionately, honestly and quickly. Of course I also wanted that same compassionate doctor to be a ruthless assassin who would gleefully kill any cancer cells that might have mistakenly infiltrated my body. Would this Dr. Kaminski be my Dr. Jekyll and Mr. Hyde?

About halfway through our visit, I mentally decided to give Dr. Kaminski the benefit of the doubt. He reminded me of television's version of yesteryear's kindly physician, a huge compliment coming from me. At the time, Alex and I hadn't a clue just how lucky we were to be sitting with one of the world's foremost lymphoma experts.

What I really wanted to know was how long I had to live—*if* I had lymphoma, although I still didn't believe that I did. Dr. Kaminski explained that there were many new treatments on the horizon, but for the type of lymphoma he suspected, the median length of life from diagnosis was currently about eight years. As I thought that simply wasn't long enough, he said he wanted me to leave his office with hope. I wanted to throw myself at his feet and beg for a guarantee that he could put me on the far side of the median. A lifetime on the far side. Hadn't the article said he had found a cure?

Dr. Kaminski wanted me to have a CT scan, and before our visit concluded, he had invited a surgeon to join us. Together they examined me and spoke "Medicalese," in which I am not fluent. I did, however, understand the two doctors to agree that a biopsy would conclusively confirm suspicions. At least I knew what a biopsy was. Dr. Chang, the surgeon, would cut me open, remove a small piece of me, a pathologist would look at it, see nothing wrong, and this little scare would end. Period.

Alex, reserved and quiet by nature, had scarcely said a

word throughout our appointment, and he said even less as we walked hand in hand to the car. Finally, I said lightly, "Hey, don't look so glum. A couple of doctors just want to carve me up a little. You know, do a little excavating. So—let's humor them and show them I'm fine, okay?"

"Okay," Alex agreed, trying to smile. "If they want to biopsy, the good news is that the doctors must not be sure you have lymphoma. Maybe they think there's a mistake, too." A year later, he would tell me that he had added silently, "But what if the biopsy confirms their suspicions? Then what?"

CHAPTER TWO
THE GREAT EXCAVATION

Several days passed before the CT scan and the "Great Excavation." My body had acquired its own forty-eight-hour rhythm. One day it stayed awake throughout the day. The next afternoon it required an hour or two nap, although require is an understatement. It was impossible to stay awake through the drowsy spells. And at night, hot flashes often plagued me, but they were nothing new.

One Saturday, after running errands, Alex and I passed a show in a convention center. He wondered if I was up to stopping in, which I was—sort of. I didn't feel like walking through the show, so I told him I would wait for him by the food court where I promptly put my head on the table and fell asleep. Forty-five minutes later, he found me there, snoozing in public. "Geez, Alex, was I snoring?"

"Just drooling," he teased.

Our family was concerned about me, and we had honestly told them everything we knew. Did we think we could diminish our own fear by spreading it around?

I routinely check email early each morning. A day or two before the CT scan, I received a message from one of our well-intentioned family members. It said, "Have been researching lymphoma. You have a 50 percent chance of survival." I stared at that computer screen for what seemed like an eternity. What? A 50 percent chance of survival? We didn't even know if I *had* lymphoma, and we certainly hadn't considered death and dying. I was furious. I wanted to reply, "Have been researching life. You have a 0 percent chance of survival."

Instead, ranting and raving, I flew into the bathroom where Alex was just getting out of the shower. "This is bull," I squawked. "Nobody has a 50 percent chance of survival. Everybody has 100 percent certainty of dying. Nobody wants to admit it. And I'll be damned if I'll let some email inform me of my odds. My odds are as good as yours— we're all gonna die from something. And lymphoma will *not* get me." I carried on about the possibility of getting hit by a truck, of living to be one hundred and dying of natural causes, of not knowing how much time any one of us has on this earth. Wrapped in a towel, Alex just stood there, arms by his sides, enduring my fury. And then, without a word, he put his arms around me. Need I say that statistics are best delivered by medical experts?

Picture Day arrived. Alex drove me to the hospital for the CT scan, stopping for gas on the way. I went into the convenience store and bought myself a raspberry Krispy Kreme doughnut with which to reward myself after the scan. We were both on edge. Summoning a smokescreen for our fears, we quibbled about which hospital entrance to use.

As we waited in the holding pen with other patients

who were equally anxious, no doubt, for their photographic sessions, the receptionist served me what I have since named the "kitty cocktail." What was that stuff, I wondered. It wasn't awful, but I'd rather have had a V-8. Okay, at that moment, I'd rather have had a margarita—and I don't drink. As I left Alex in the reception area, I quipped over my shoulder, "I'll tell them to get my good side. Shall we order the 8x10's or the wallets?" He didn't even smile.

My first glimpse of the machine reminded me of the doughnut waiting out in the car. There was a big hole through which I would slide while the machine snapped pictures of my innards. But first I was served another kitty cocktail and poked with an IV so that iodine, a dye, could pour through my body and help whoever was looking to better see whatever it was he or she wanted to see. No one warned me I would taste the iodine. Bon appetit.

With the liquids in the proper recesses of my body, I lay on my back to await the photography. As a mechanical voice filled the room, instructing me when to breathe in and when to breathe out, I noticed the manufacturer's label on the machine—GE—and I started silently singing its jingle, "We bring good things to life." Then I changed it to "We help good things to live." That was it—I would live! GE wouldn't let me do otherwise. Just as the taste of iodine flooded my mouth, there was a whole corporation making sure I was healthy! I could hardly wait to get out of that doughnut and eat the one waiting for me.

The following day, I gave some thought to the word lymphoma. There was brain cancer. Breast cancer. Prostate cancer. Lung cancer. Liver cancer. Bone cancer. *They* were bad because every one of them actually included the word cancer. I decided that I should be worried if lymphoma were called lymphoma cancer. But it wasn't. Unattached to the C-word, lymphoma couldn't be too bad.

I even halved lymphoma into lymph and oma. Lymph rhymed with nymph, and oma was a German word for grandmother. Accordingly, I envisioned hundreds of sweet, geriatric fairies happily flying through forests protecting every living thing. I began, ever so slowly, to admit the possibility of having "nymphoma," and how bad could that be, given the meaning I had attached to it? I even put Alex on performance notice in case I became a nymphomaniac. He was unamused by my mockery of a serious disease, but ah, denial and mirth are fabulous stress suppressors.

I was also certain that I was emotionally equipped for the challenge *if* I had nymphoma. After all, I had faced adversity before. Several years earlier, my world had instantly changed when my former husband had decided one day to drop out of life. Any security, financial or otherwise, I had ever thought I had was completely obliterated. Among other things, the IRS was not amused that he had failed to pay our income taxes, and I was left to clean up the mess. Four years and lots of hard work later, I had resolved matters and started over, albeit battered and bruised and convinced that the IRS was a masterpiece of bureaucracy and redundancy.

And there was the time that two teenage gang members had tried to gun me down in broad daylight for no reason at all. I had simply been driving down the street in a perfectly decent part of West Palm Beach when they had emptied their weapons. In an instant, my car had been badly injured, but I'd been unharmed—at least physically. Several months later, I had walked away from that fiasco convinced that the justice system was a masterpiece of hypocrisy. Why else would they lock up juries and set criminals free?

Yes sirree, I knew what it was like for life to change in an instant. I knew how to handle adversity. I knew what it was like to be up and to be down, emotionally and financially. I knew how to face cold, impersonal bureaucratic agencies, and I was still certain—no matter how nice Dr. Kaminski and Judy had been—that the health care system was just another bureaucracy. Surely no one would care whether I ended up running a marathon or being turned over in some bed like a piece of meat on a rotisserie. I'd had experience, I told myself, and could cope with any challenge. I am woman. Hear me roar. Little did I know how quickly my roar would dwindle to a whimper.

Excavation Day arrived on January 30. Alex and I left for the hospital before dawn on a cold, dark, snowy morning. My spirits were high because I was determined to believe that this test would conclusively prove that I was fine. And I was willing to be drugged and knifed to prove it. Wasn't I the martyr?

At outpatient surgery, I changed into the hospital's mandatory uniform, a one-size-fits-all hospital gown which, I was quite sure, was designed to reduce individuals to one-description-fits-all: patient. Deprived of individuality, how easy then to further reduce patients to a record of symptoms. I wanted to tell the hospital that one size does *not* fit all, and that patients surely have different color preferences as well. I rambled on to Alex that Calvin Klein could do wonders for these blah uniforms. Surely he would use different colors, and of course he would make them in different sizes. There would be long ones for tall people who had to contend with near-indecent exposure, as well as whatever illness afflicted them. And there would be small ones for small people who struggled to keep their oversized uniforms on. No hospital, I complained, would ever act on the suggestion of offering its patients small, medium, and large sizes and a choice of colors, but doing so might make us feel a little more human.

An IV was inserted into my arm, and I began to get a little sleepy. Alex kissed me as I was wheeled away. I was sorry that this was taking time from his busy schedule, but it would all be over soon.

In the operating room, the temperature felt like an Antarctic winter day. One nurse fastened my legs to the table while two others stretched out and strapped down my left arm perpendicular to my body. Looking up at everyone, it suddenly seemed so bizarre that I had allowed myself to be drugged and clamped to a metal table surrounded by strangers wielding knives. "What's wrong with this picture?" was my last thought.

Still in the operating room, I awoke. The overhead lights were bright, and people seemed to be scurrying around the room. I asked Dr. Chang if he would show me what he had removed, and he placed a small vial before my sleepy eyes.

Floating in it was what looked like a bloody pea.

At that moment, I realized the significance of The Pea. It would determine my future. The Pea knew whether or not I would live to dance at my grandchildren's weddings. The Pea knew whether or not I would grow old along with Alex. Who was going to look at that bloody pea and interpret just what it had to say? Somebody I had never even met? Somebody who didn't know how much I wanted to live? Somebody who had maybe just had a fight with his wife? I wanted to bolt off that operating table and hand deliver that bloody pea to the pathologist. I wanted to look him or her in the eye and beg, "This belongs to me. It's the key to my life. Please, oh please, let me live."

It occurred to me that I would be placing blind faith in people I didn't know if I had this disease. There would be people who would interpret X-rays, CT scans, and who knew what else. Lying there on the table, I panicked, wondering if these people realized how profoundly their reports impact people's lives. I desperately needed to meet these invisible prognosticators and to plead with them to remember that I, like them, am a human being with hopes and dreams and a family. But of course I couldn't meet any of them. I simply had to place my faith in their experience and my hope in their perfection. Though I am ordinarily a trusting soul, we were talking about my life here, and I felt so vulnerable by having no choice but to place blind trust in people into whose eyes I could not see.

And just how would blood tests, CT scans, or biopsies measure my emotions? Would the pathologist reading the bloody pea also calculate my fear? Would he send a report to Dr. Kaminski that said Mrs. de Parry has such and such stage of lymphoma—and by the way, her fear factor is off the charts? Of course not. The medical experts would be interested only in the parts of me that they could put into test tubes and vials or see under microscopes, on slides, or on film. I wanted to scream, "But that's only a little part of me! Don't forget the important parts—the ones that make me laugh and cry and love." I doubted anyone would have listened to that plea.

I was the first to return to the recovery room, which was large and empty except for Alex. I was so happy to see him. What had he been thinking while I was away? He wouldn't say, but he held my hand tightly. Months later, Alex would confide that he had worried about a stranger cutting into me while he sat isolated and unable to protect me should anything go wrong during the surgery. He also hoped that there had been a mix-up, but began to prepare himself for the possibility that I may in fact have lymphoma. Still, he convinced himself that it couldn't possibly be so bad, since I neither looked nor acted sick. Sure, he had noticed the lethargy, but he'd also noticed signs of improvement. Even if this biopsy showed some kind of lymphoma, he told himself that—*if* we had to—we would deal with this quickly and go on with our lives.

A nurse explained that I could return home when my vital signs had stabilized and I had urinated. As she helped me to the bathroom, IV pole in tow, I couldn't help but think how ridiculous I must look shuffling across the room in nonskid socks and a gown that ten of me could fit into. Topping this ensemble was the paper hat hiding all my hair. And forbidden as I was to wear my contacts, my makeup-less face was covered in large part by my old, ugly glasses. Not exactly power clothes.

I hated for Alex to see me this way. Sure, he saw me every morning at my worst, but this was worse than my worst. The very surroundings, the IV pole, the absurd outfit—all stripped away the me we knew. If I could just find my funny face, Alex would recognize the old me. As I exited the bathroom, he sat across the room at my bedside, hunched on the edge of a chair, pulling his wedding ring up to his knuckle and pushing it back again. I put on a big grin, took the IV pole in both hands and began to twirl around with my new dance partner, Mr. I. V. Pole. Alex jumped to his feet and ran toward me, mumbling something about falling. "Oh Alex, you need to lighten up and have a little fun," I teased. Again, he didn't smile.

I had endured fever and general malaise for a month, and I began to look for any sign of increasing energy. I had not met my own expectations during the month of January, and my frustration was escalating. Lying on the couch for hours on end, taking naps, running fevers, and spending time having medical tests left little time to accomplish what I had set out to do. Alex, who has always given himself more tasks every day than anyone can possibly complete, was doing his job and mine, and this became an increasing source of worry for me, not to mention guilt. When I returned home from the Great Excavation, I determined that I must make up in February what I had failed to do in January. I'd completed the medical tests, and this nightmare would soon be over. I was sure of it.

CHAPTER THREE
THE QUEEN OF DENIAL

A few days after the CT scan and biopsy, Alex and I waited in the examining room for the results, which we still hoped would indicate that nothing was wrong. Our hope waned in an instant when Dr. Kaminski reported that the CT scan and biopsy confirmed low-grade, follicular, small-cleaved lymphoma, grade I, non-Hodgkin's, stage IV. What a mouthful—and what a bad spin on a little fever that had broken four weeks earlier.

My white blood counts were soaring. Dr. Kaminski discussed various treatment options should my counts continue to rise. "Watch and wait," a period when no treatment is administered, was probably not an option for long, he stated. When he mentioned chemotherapy, all I heard was the sound of vomiting. He talked about clinical trials. His Bexxar was still under FDA review, so his magic cure was as yet unavailable. He was clearly moving me in a direction I did not want to take. But with false bravado, I joked to him, "Well, let's fix this fast. Dead salesmen don't usually meet their quotas, and my boss might get upset." Dr. Kaminski smiled. Alex was horrified. The wisecrack kept me from sobbing.

From the moment we left the examining room until we arrived in the lobby, my eyes stared straight down at my feet. There was a lump the size of a basketball in my throat, and I knew I would cry if I looked up at anyone, particularly Alex. We had met at the hospital, and he asked if I would like to go with him and return for my car later. "No," I mumbled. "I'm okay." He knew I wasn't, and he put his arm around me. I buried my head in his shoulder and cried, "I just wanted Dr. Kaminski to say everything was okay. I want this to go away and leave us alone."

Tears flowed gently down my cheeks. Alex put his other arm around me and drew me closer to him, as if his embrace could fix what Dr. Kaminski couldn't. "Whatever happens," he said, "we'll get through this."

"How do you know that?" I asked.

"Because I know *us*," he replied, wiping my tears away.

Silently, I wondered if I had just been handed a death sentence, but I pulled myself together and assured Alex I was fine. In fact, I told him I was going to stop at one of our favorite antique stores and then head home to start dinner.

I did stop at the antique store. I usually loved rummaging for bargains, but on that day, I wandered through all three floors of the store without ever noticing a single item. All I could think about was lymphoma. Cancer. Chemotherapy. Clinical trials. Alex. Juli. What would happen to our lives?

I told myself that test results can be skewed. Surely there was an acceptable arbitrary margin of error. Or maybe this was just bad feng shui. Could my chakras be clogged?

Had Dr. Kaminski confused me with someone else? It was much too soon to surrender to scientific "facts," I thought. Talk about grasping at straws.

Alex, on the other hand, would later explain that he promptly hunkered down for a long haul. He immediately refused to indulge in what-ifs, and he saw the futility of expending energy on wishing that cancer wasn't here. It was, and so he consciously asked himself what he could do to mitigate the disruption in our lives. Knowing that he would be of no help to me if he allowed himself to crumble, he resolved to stay focused on a positive outcome and to safeguard our optimistic attitudes—which he believed were absolutely critical to the ultimate goal of wellness. He saw that we would be spending more and more time at the hospital and that managing his time would be more critical than ever. He promised himself he would assume my job when necessary and learn how to juggle medical appointments, work, and whatever else would give me the mental energy to heal. Deliberately, he appointed himself Head Cheerleader, although it would take me months to notice.

I had promised to call Juli after our appointment. By the time I wandered through the antique store, I had pulled myself together enough to do so. Sitting in my car in the parking lot, I dialed her number and hoped that I could sound strong and brave. I think—I hope—that I did. I told her there were several clinical trials I could enter, that there was great hope for a cure and that, yes, this was one big royal pain, but I would be fine. I tried to sound as hopeful and cheerful as I possibly could. What I really felt was that

I was the child and she the mother. All I really wanted was to collapse in her arms and tell her how much I loved her. But she was twelve hundred miles away, and there was nothing she could do.

Next, I stopped by the office. Alex wasn't expecting me, and I found him sitting at my desk wearing a mask of fear on his face, clearly visible for the first time, at least to me. Across from him sat Greta, his eighteen-year-old daughter, weeping. She rose, walked the few steps toward me, and put her arms around me. I assured her things would be fine, that this was just a little bump in the road of life. Somehow I managed to keep my composure, although the look I had seen on Alex's face nearly shattered it.

At dinner that evening, we told Zan, Alex's thirteen-year-old son who lives with us most of the time. Although Alex and I had not discussed in any great detail how we would handle a real illness, we had both agreed to maintain as normal a life as possible. We briefly explained the illness to Zan and assured him we would not allow this to affect his normal routine. Thirteen-year-old boys have much better things to think about than their wicked stepmothers' problems, and Zan took the news in stride. Like his father, he never turns a problem into a crisis.

When I told my sister Karen, I felt obliged to keep the conversation as light as possible in order to alleviate her fears. Humor, I believe, allows us to avoid staring directly at adversity, and I had always used it to masquerade my own fears. Wisecracks had, in fact, often kept me from falling to pieces.

My sisters Nancy and Karen were sixteen and thirteen respectively when I was born, the result, I suspect, of an amorous accident. Both Nancy, who had died eleven years earlier, and Karen had voluptuous bodies. I have always been flat, straight, and skinny. They were endowed with large melons. I received pancakes. Since puberty, when it became clear that my pancakes would never grow into melons, they had teased me unmercifully. It was time to get Karen back.

When I called her, I excitedly told her that all the reports were back. I'd seen them with my own eyes, and all the radiologists, pathologists, and doctors had referred to my swollen lymph nodes as *breasts*. Yes, in print, the word I had always wanted attributed to me was there—*breasts*, not chest. Medical science had finally proven that I do indeed have melons, however underdeveloped. Karen giggled as I had wanted her to, and it set the tone for the truth.

I lay awake in the darkness much of that night. Listening to Alex's quiet, steady breathing, I grieved for him. He hadn't bargained for this. I reminisced about falling in love with him. Initially, our romance had been complicated by the twelve hundred miles between us, as well as by the scars from our previous marriages. But eventually, we'd become the best of friends because, I thought, we simply balanced and completed each other.

I'd often laughed that we should be the poster couple for Opposites Attract. He's serious. I'm playful. He's a conversational minimalist, saying in two words what it would take me twenty sentences to say. While he withholds his thoughts and feelings, I easily divulge what is on my mind, at least to a few people. While he's the pragmatist, I'm the romantic. He's a workaholic while I wonder why he makes no time to enjoy a movie. While he remains calm through anything and everything, my emotions rise high and fall low. Sometimes I'd teased him, "You alive under all that composure?"

I worried that Alex was much too stoic to cope with a major illness. I was afraid that he had no idea how to reach out for help, and that he would try to appear as strong and emotionless about this situation as he was about everything else. Through his fifty-four years, he and his small family had been blessed with excellent health. His mother Lisa, at eighty-three, and his father Ted, at eighty-nine, still lived in their own home not far from ours, walked five miles a day, drove themselves wherever they wanted to go, wintered in Florida, and suffered not a single ailment. Alex had never endured the day-to-day agonies of illness, much less the loss of a close family member. He couldn't have a clue what to expect.

On the other hand, I knew from experience that a major illness wreaks havoc because I grew up surrounded by it. When I was six, my mother's mother became blind and bedridden. Since she was a Christian Scientist, we never learned the cause. As a child, I knew only that my mother spent her days in my grandmother's room caring for her. When I was twelve, my father's mother became bedridden and moved in with us. My mother could not manage the care of both grandmothers, so my parents hired a live-in nurse to help. She hated kids. I hated her back. I was no longer permitted to have friends over because our childish noises might have disturbed my grandmothers, or so my parents thought. Never mind that I made ear-splitting mistakes practicing the piano. I never could figure out how the noise my friends and I made could have been worse.

For almost as far back as I can remember until almost the time I left for college, illness had dictated every move our family had made, and I had hated that. I had vowed that when I grew up, I would never, ever let any illness dominate my life or the life of my family. So far it hadn't, but would that soon change? I cringed at the thought.

Lying in bed that night, I thought, too, about losing someone you love. Alex hadn't faced that experience, but years earlier I had lost my father and my sister. I recalled Daddy's illness, a stroke that had immobilized his body and nearly destroyed his speech. At the time, I was a grown woman who loved her father dearly, but those old childhood scars had resurfaced, and I had hated being around illness again, especially illness that claimed someone I loved so dearly.

I did, however, recognize the indignities that Daddy suffered during the year between his stroke and his death. His sharp lawyer's mind was trapped in a broken shell, and though he never surrendered his sense of humor, he despised his helplessness. *That* I understood, and I had secretly hoped that I would just drop dead one day. I doubted that the Invisible Invader would give me that luxury.

I wondered how Alex and Juli would feel if they had to watch me waste away as I had watched Daddy. Far away and entrenched with her own family and job, Juli at least would be spared the daily agonies. But how would Alex cope? Would they feel as helpless as I did when I had wanted to fix Daddy and had driven myself half crazy when I couldn't? Neither Alex nor Juli had probably ever considered the fact that I would not always be around, and I wondered how much they depended on me, and for what. Until Daddy's illness, I had never realized how much I depended on him for a million little things, and I still missed our lively conversations. Would Alex and Juli miss talking with me as much as I still missed talking with Daddy?

My thoughts shifted to my sister Nancy. She was fifty-nine and perfectly healthy when she got up one morning, had a stroke, and was comatose by lunch. When I saw her in the hospital, my beautiful, glamorous sister had become nearly indistinguishable from the sheets. Honoring a decision she had made much earlier, my brother-in-law and nephews stopped life support the day after her stroke. Moments later, she died as I held her hand. I ached with sadness when I walked away from her down the long hospital corridor. That was one walk I fervently hoped Alex and Juli would never have to make, but my mind and body were clearly out of sync, the latter obviously not caring for them in the least.

I had never reconciled whether prolonged illness or sudden death was easier to bear. Selfishly, I was glad that my father had given us that extra year after his stroke, but it was painfully hard on him. And knowing of his impending death made it no easier to accept when it finally came. What

I did know was that illness and death were stressful and sad and time-consuming. Alex didn't. How could I possibly explain to him that he was in for an emotional roller coaster ride? I finally fell asleep that night promising myself to talk with him about this.

The following morning, I begged Alex not to try to carry this burden alone. This was not the time for his disciplined stoicism. Stress, I reminded him, destroys our bodies, and he was already on stress overload without this challenge. I told him that I was afraid his health was as much at risk as mine if he were to internalize his feelings about this illness as much as he did about everything else. I pleaded with him not to let the Invisible Invader destroy him, and I suggested that he learn somehow to express his emotions to me or to anyone who would listen. Since he said little as I spoke, I virtually delivered a monologue. Was he listening, I wondered?

I forgot to tell Alex that I wasn't ready to reveal our misfortune to anyone outside of our family. Although I had encouraged him to express his emotions, he's ordinarily such a private person that I guess I never thought he would say much to anyone. I certainly didn't know yet how to respond to other people, and I did not want to hear, "Oh, you poor thing."

After all, lymphoma wasn't happening to me. Even though I had spoken and thought of it, I still felt that I had been speaking or thinking of someone else. I found it impossible to believe that such an insidious disease would dare to interrupt our lives. Surely other facts would surface and disprove the findings. Yes, I wore a cloak of delusion, and it fit quite nicely, thank you very much.

Within days of our conversation, flowers began to arrive at our home, clearly because Alex had heeded my advice about sharing his feelings and had divulged our predicament. I was relieved that he was opening up and thought that it was healthy for him to verbalize, if not his feelings, at least the situation, and I took comfort in knowing that he would learn from others who had experienced similar situations. It never occurred to me that Alex—being Alex—was hardly looking for support. He was searching for specific answers from anyone who had faced the disease. He wanted to know what they had done—and where.

Within days of launching his fact-finding mission, we had more flowers than I knew what to do with. At the risk of sounding ungrateful and never receiving flowers again, our house was beginning to look like a morgue. Of course I appreciated the sentiments from each and every sender, and I was deeply touched by the outpouring of good wishes from all the wonderful people who knew nothing else to do. But just who were they sending all these flowers to, anyway? It couldn't be me. I wanted nothing to remind me that our lives were any different than they had always been.

Worse, I couldn't bear to watch the flowers shrivel and die. Each death reminded me how short life is, and I feared that I, too, might quickly be discarded. After about a week of receiving bouquets, I gave subsequent arrivals away in order to avoid witnessing their speedy demise. Fortunately, one friend sent a plant, and I nurtured it throughout my entire illness.

Alex, too, began to do things he normally wouldn't do. Dragging him out on weeknights was about as easy as extracting teeth from a live alligator. He was too busy reviewing paperwork from the office. Every night. And he'd never been able to pull off a surprise. But early in February, when he told me not to plan anything for a particular Tuesday evening, he delighted me with dinner at a charming restaurant followed by a performance of *Phantom of the Opera*.

Soon after, on another weeknight, we enjoyed the St. Petersburg Symphony Orchestra, which played some of my favorite music. I couldn't help but close my eyes and wonder if we'd ever see that beautiful city—together. We'd certainly hoped to—someday.

Everyone else seemed to be taking this far more seriously than I, perhaps because I knew so little about lymphoma. Or perhaps because I was still not completely convinced that I had it. Even if I did, I desperately wanted to believe that something would deliver me from it at the last minute. And I wondered how in the world I had ever gotten into this mess.

After all, I'd always been so healthy. Despite the fact that I had taken better care of my car than my body—and that's not saying much—my body and I had always lived in perfect symbiosis. I'd nourished it adequately but not especially admirably. I hadn't exercised it regularly, but neither did I live a sedentary life. The only serious medical procedure I ever had was a partial hysterectomy in 1978, which at that time was the common remedy when Pap smears indicated suspicious cells. Otherwise, I'd breezed through life absolutely fine. At least until the previous two and a half years.

In the summer of 1999, my body started its rebellion. In July of that year, I yawned during dinner one evening. My mother, who was visiting us, asked, "Honey, why are you so tired?"

"Oh, it's nothing. I just woke up several times last night. I was so hot."

"Why, Honey, you're having night sweats. You're just going through menopause."

Alex was so embarrassed that the color drained from his face. I was dumbfounded—menopause? Suddenly I remembered that the doctor who had yanked out my uterus all those years ago had warned me that I might have menopausal symptoms. Hmm. Maybe I should see a gynecologist. Hadn't been to one in twenty-one years.

The gynecologist "confirmed" menopause, and quickly wrote a prescription for hormone replacement therapy without taking any time to address my concerns about it. In September, I returned for the follow-up visit and another blood test. The hormones weren't reducing the symptoms, so I quit taking them after another three or four months and never returned to the gynecologist. The symptoms just weren't bothersome enough, and I just laughed off the hot flashes as power surges.

The following summer, my body again reminded me that it needed some attention when the balls of my feet started to hurt periodically and the joints across the tops of my toes occasionally swelled. I'd always ignored little aches and pains, but these weren't so little. Alex and I could only suppose that our stairs were the culprit. My office was on the second floor, our stairs were oak, and I flew barefooted up and down many times during the day, taking two stairs at a time, landing on the balls of my feet with each step. I began to take the stairs flat-footed, one at a time, and even wore cushioned shoes, all the while joking about becoming an old lady. Nothing helped, and it was no joke. Sometimes those stairs felt like Mt. Everest as I climbed them. Whatever was going on, I didn't like it.

In March 2001, I saw a rheumatologist who gave me about sixty seconds of his time, during which he told me I had rheumatoid arthritis. He added that it wasn't a "classic" case because it only affected my feet, and he said that I should take methotrexate and have weekly blood tests. He handed me the prescription and a couple of brochures and left the room as quickly as he had entered.

When I read the brochures, I discovered that methotrexate is a form of chemotherapy that can damage other organs, and that the weekly blood tests would monitor for damage. That wasn't exactly what I had in mind. I wanted to know the underlying cause and how it could be fixed, but I never could get that answer. I reluctantly began the medication and underwent the weekly pokes. The medicine made me feel weak, tired, and slightly nauseated. My feet still hurt. The cure was worse than the cause. I wanted to know other options, but I got no answers. Within weeks, I quit the methotrexate.

By early summer, I found another doctor who took a much broader view of rheumatoid arthritis. He agreed that I did not have a classic case of the disease, and felt that nutritional changes could possibly keep me off drugs. I eliminated all forms of dairy products from my diet and made other minor changes.

My feet really did improve. They weren't pain free all the time, but the improvement was significant. I was pleased that my body was cooperating. I was too young to be getting old, I told myself, and I was glad that my body and I were at peace again. At least I thought we were, until that fever in December interrupted my sense of security.

In January 2002, after I was diagnosed with lymphoma, I retrieved a copy of the September 1999 blood test and there—in bold print—was my lymphocyte count. *High*, it said, in big, bold letters. I stared at the paper for a very long time, feeling betrayed by a female doctor who—if she had bothered to read the report—might not have blown me off as another casualty of middle-aged menopause.

And was the improvement in my feet merely coincidental? Intuition had often told me that my hot flashes were not menopausal and that the pain and swelling in my feet were not caused by rheumatoid arthritis, but it had never occurred to me that I was on a collision course with cancer. How was I to know that hot flashes were symptomatic of lymphoma or that the pain and inflammation in my feet were signs of my immune system shorting out? That obviously didn't occur to the three doctors I saw either. It would take a third-year emergency room resident—Dr. Ketcham—to take the time to ask questions, to listen to my history, and to fit the puzzle together.

It's no wonder Dr. Kaminski had to earn my trust. It's not that I didn't want to trust him. I did, but it would take some time for me to recognize that he and his staff treated patients and paperwork without the hasty indifference that I had come to assume was standard practice. From the beginning, he and Judy seemed to care about my cancer *and* about the rest of me. They also gave me copies of every report from every test I had. Even though I didn't have a clue what most of the words meant, the message was clear: we have nothing to hide from you, and we want you to be informed about your disease. What a concept, I thought. And not only did they give me copies, but by phone, email, or during an appointment, Judy and Dr. Kaminski reported and interpreted test results very quickly. That meant they had actually looked at those reports. It was amazing, I thought, that they seemed to know the importance of trust.

Still, by the end of February 2002, when our home looked and smelled like a morgue and Dr. Kaminski was convinced that the Invisible Invader had attacked, I wanted to argue with the entire medical community that the test results were wrong. My body was telling me a different story than what the reports were telling them. My energy was returning, and I felt fine. I was willing to concede that there may be an aberrant deviation of normal cells, but I wanted to suggest that it was the result of some undiscovered vitamin deficiency.

How could the test results possibly belong to someone who was back at work and feeling perfectly well? And how in the world would I find time to accomplish everything I needed to accomplish if I had to continue going to the hospital all the time? My day planner had no room for *any* internal malfunction. If I just ignored it, would it all go away?

For nearly two months, I was the queen of denial. Oh, I'd wept briefly a couple of times, mainly out of frustration, but never because I believed I was staring a life-threatening disease squarely in the face. I mostly joked about it. Alex and I had few conversations about lymphoma, and those were not only brief, but also limited mostly to the schedule of appointments. Besides the one monologue I had delivered encouraging him to express his emotions, we had avoided serious discussions—which was exactly the way I wanted it. I never did take my own advice very well.

CHAPTER FOUR

BIG GIRLS *DO* CRY

One afternoon in late February, I was on my way home from meeting with clients when the word "cancer" seemed to scream from a news program on the radio, to which I had not been paying particular attention. How dare that radio remind me of cancer? Angrily, I changed the station, only to hear the song "Big Girls Don't Cry." Suddenly I started screaming back at the radio, "Oh yes, they *do* cry!" And with that, a torrent of tears gushed forth so hard that I couldn't see to drive. Fortunately, I was close to a cul-de-sac where homes were under construction but where no one yet lived. I pulled to the end of the street, stopped my car, and let it all out. I sobbed so hard my whole body shook like a tree in a hurricane. I pounded the steering wheel until my hands hurt. I screamed and cursed and cried out, "Please let me live! Please. Please. Please."

For the first time in my life, a mixture of raw fear, grief, and anger gripped me. A thousand thoughts that I had been repressing for nearly two months rushed at me at once. Would I live to enjoy my grandchildren? Would I live to see them graduate from college? Would I grow old with Alex?

I'd counted on many years together, and I grieved at the possible loss of anything less than a long lifetime with him.

And what had I ever done that really mattered? At least Alex's homes were standing testimony to a lifetime of work, but what would *I* leave behind? Who would keep the marketing materials I had written? Who would remember the countless hours I had spent helping clients choose a floorplan, a kitchen sink, a bathroom tile?

Would I become deformed and emaciated? How much pain would there be? Would I become bedridden like my grandmothers? I couldn't bear the thought. If I couldn't enjoy life, contribute to it, and remain independent, I didn't want to stick around.

But I *did* want to stick around. How could this be happening? I'd been able to solve some difficulties in my life, but I had no control over *this*. How would I confront the reality of this predicament? Oh dear Lord, I prayed, I'll give up anything if You'll find the grace and goodness to return my health. Looking toward the heavens, I told God I would do *anything* He wanted and begged Him to give me a sign.

After what seemed like hours but was probably several long minutes, my body quit heaving and the tears dried up. I could just hear Daddy reminding me, "When the going gets tough, the tough get going," and I tried to persuade myself that this was tough, but I was tougher. Silently at first, then out loud, I began to chant, "I can beat this. I can beat this. I can beat this."

There in the car, I had a long talk with myself about

the power of positive thinking and the strength of the human spirit. "Mind over matter," my Christian Scientist grandmother had preached. "Never give up," said Winston Churchill. Then Cervantes reminded me, "The man who is prepared has his battle half fought," and I knew what I had to do. I would learn everything I possibly could about the Invisible Invader. I would take the offensive, defy the odds, the probabilities, and the medians—and I would *win*. By the time I finally headed home, I was fiercely and passionately ready to tackle whatever was necessary to learn about my enemy.

I've always needed to know where I'm going, whether it's on a trip or to a meeting. When it came to important things, I never was very good at winging it. Now life itself had blindsided me, and I faced its biggest crisis without preparation. I wasn't even sure how to prepare for this catastrophe. But I had resolved to confront the Invisible Invader with as much energy and passion as I had ever devoted to anything.

That was easier said than done. I'd spent my adult life helping people buy and plan their new homes. Nothing exactly scientific about that. In fact, nothing I had ever done required any knowledge of science. Things just worked, and at the risk of sounding intellectually apathetic, I was never particularly curious as to why. I'm sure I was born without a left brain. When the Invisible Invader came calling, I regretted having paid so little attention to science. Cells. Proteins. DNA. Lymphocytes. What were their functions? Was I the dimmest light bulb in the chandelier?

I needed a crash course in "Lymphoma for Dummies." Why hadn't someone written that book? Without its existence, just how was I to learn everything I needed to know? At least I had the presence of mind to realize that Dr. Kaminski's and Judy's roles were to treat my disease, not to be my personal Lymphoma 101 tutors. I had nowhere to turn but to Alex. He would be my science expert. He's much more well-rounded than I am. He has both sides of his brain, and he uses them. Whether it's physics or history, music or economics, he has a natural curiosity for all living and nonliving subjects, and he has the memory of an elephant. Best of all, he graduated *pre-med!* Surely he would have no trouble understanding this disease, its causes and its cures. Mentally, I designated Alex to figure this whole thing out and explain lymphoma in simple terms to me.

What was I thinking? Alex definitely has his good points, but he explains everything on a postdoctorate level, using as few words as possible. Clearly, he was not the person to ask for simple explanations, but I did. As questions came to me over the next few days, I fired them off faster than a machine gun. Alex, what's a cell? Alex, explain DNA. Alex, I thought protein was something you ate. Alex, what's a lymphocyte? Alex, explain the lymph system. Alex, Alex, Alex . . . I drove him crazy with questions.

I begged him to answer each question as if he were talking to a five-year-old. Draw me a picture. Use simple words and analogies. He would try. I would then ask a question in response to his explanation. He'd try again. I'd ask another question. Soon he was off somewhere in left field as far as I was concerned. Frustrated, I would complain, "Alex, you're too intelligent for your own good. And certainly for mine." His unfathomable answers were making my brain feel feeble. Worse, my education was at a standstill.

I'd been asking all these questions whenever they popped into my mind. In the kitchen. On the way to a meeting. When he was standing in the middle of a construction site with saws and nailguns drowning out my voice. I suggested that if we just sat down one evening, we could accomplish more. Alex agreed, so I put together questions and notes. On the dining room table, I spread out the booklets and pamphlets we had gathered and even brought out the encyclopedias.

I wanted Alex to start at the beginning, to explain a cell and how it functions. He began. I wasn't getting it. Having always learned well from visual aids, I began to draw what I thought he was saying. No, that wasn't right, he said. Well, draw it for me, I replied. Alex isn't an artist. We kept going. I still didn't quite grasp the cell concept, but I went on to DNA, knowing that lymphoma had something to do with a flaw in the DNA.

"Alex, could you explain just what DNA is?"

"It's deoxyribonucleic acid," he answered. Like that told me a lot.

"And just what does it do?" I asked.

"It chemically writes each person's genetic program," he answered, as if I were supposed to understand that little tidbit of information.

"And just what does that mean, and what does it have

to do with lymphoma?" I questioned.

Alex is normally unflappable, but he flapped. One of his eyebrows cocked, his jaw squared, his voice dropped, he looked straight at me, and said, "Betsy, you're not asking for a crash course. You're trying to go to graduate school without the basics." Then he rose from the chair and took a couple of steps toward the kitchen before turning around and adding, "Scientists were just figuring out the significance of DNA when I was in college, and that was more than thirty years ago." And then he walked out of the room.

I had pushed Alex to his limit. Hadn't I always known that if I wanted a simple answer, Alex was not the person from whom to get it? Worse, he'd remembered that college was so many years ago. Not only had our conversation made him recognize the inadequacy of his teaching skills, but it had also reminded him of his age. And just maybe he was having difficulty adjusting to the idea of the Invisible Invader. Maybe he thought I was the stupidest person alive. I felt horrible. To the very best of his abilities, he really had tried.

That night, I sat at the dining room table studying the pamphlets and encyclopedias until after two o'clock in the morning. I drew circles to represent cells and wrote their different parts in the circles. My drawings looked like a five-year-old's, but they were the visual aids I needed to help me understand and remember what I was learning.

There was the nucleus of the cell wherein DNA lies tightly coiled, holding twenty-three pairs of chromosomes and a couple of thousand genes. DNA holds the master plan for each cell's form and function, and determines the proteins it produces. Proteins are not just beef or chicken, but substances which speed up chemical reactions, as in the case of hormones, or which fight infection, as in the case of antibodies.

That night, I was reminded that DNA must be copied before cells divide. It stretches out, looking like strings of beads, each bead representing a gene. When it copies itself, it should make an exact copy. Sometimes things go wrong. In the case of follicular lymphoma, the fourteenth and eighteenth genes get crossed during reproduction, and this leads to the production of a protein called BCL2 which tells the new cells, "Don't die." I still didn't understand why it was bad to have too many cells, but I was feeling more comfortable with the concept of a single cell. I probably should have relied on my own ability to learn something before putting Alex through all those questions, I thought. Hadn't I promised myself to rely on my own strength?

I turned next to the types of cells, beginning with stem cells. Despite the controversy surrounding stem cell research in recent years, I had paid little attention. That night I discovered that cells manufactured in the bone marrow are called stem cells in their infancy. They are just baby cells waiting for genetic information to give them their specialty. So far, this was pretty easy.

So, there were two sources of new cells. One came from cell division, the other from stem cells. And the stem cells, I discovered, grew up to become one of two kinds: hematopoietic or lymphocytic cells. The hematopoietic cells would further become one of six kinds of cells: red cells, basophils, neutrophils, monocytes, eosinophils, or platelets. The lymphocytic cells would become T lymphocytes, B lymphocytes, or natural killer cells. These lymphocytic cells were also produced in the lymph nodes.

Normally, all these cells do their jobs, reproduce, and die in a predictable and orderly cycle. Cancer cells do the wrong job, divide too rapidly, and are immortal. Fortunately, they are stupid—which is why many drugs can outsmart them.

In order for the body to function properly, I learned that there was a normal range of each type of cell in the blood. A blood test called a complete blood count, or CBC, told the doctors if there were too few or too many of one kind of cell or another. A machine simply counted the number of each cell type in a certain amount of blood. Ah, I was learning.

Confident that I had completed my self-taught crash course in cellular biology, I turned to the articles and pamphlets we had gathered about lymphoma. I had whined to Alex that they contained incomprehensible words and concepts, and I'd complained that even their names were threatening. "What You Need to Know About Non-Hodgkin's Lymphoma" should have been dubbed "What Someone Else Needs to Know About Non-Hodgkin's Lymphoma." "Chemotherapy and You" should have been entitled "Chemotherapy and Some Other Poor Soul." That night, sitting at the dining room table long after Alex had gone to bed, I opened my mind and read every booklet and article we had gathered.

Still, lymphoma is a very difficult disease to understand without some scientific background. Each patient's disease presents itself and behaves differently. There are indolent and aggressive forms and thirty or so different subcategories. Mine was of the indolent nature, which to me simply meant that it was too slow or too lazy to kill me immediately. It was also circulating in my bloodstream, and even with my limited knowledge, I knew that blood circulated to every organ and tissue. By the time I finally went to bed, I couldn't help but wonder if I was just one big blob of cancer. But I also could hardly wait to recite all the details of my new knowledge to Alex.

The following morning, we stood in the kitchen and I excitedly showed him my pictures. With my hands on my hips and a sheepish grin on my face, I pranced around the kitchen island rapidly rattling off every bit of information I could remember. Alex tried not to laugh, but his amusement was quite apparent. Talking about anything scientific was so out of character for me, and we did, in fact, have quite a good laugh. I told him not to worry about understanding the more recent DNA discoveries. As the new science expert of the household, I'd catch up on them and fill him in. Sure, he chuckled, as he put his arms around me.

We had less than two weeks before our next visit with Dr. Kaminski, and I felt like a college kid facing the biggest exam of my life. I scoured the internet and found it strewn with cancer sites, but I had no idea how to judge the veracity of the material or the relevance it may or may not have to me. I thus approached the information with some skepticism. Voraciously, I re-read everything I had attempted to read earlier, and I began to comprehend more.

Alex also became much better at answering questions—or had I just become better at listening? It was probably a combination of both. Alex would months later tell me that he had genuinely wanted to answer my questions, but had initially been frustrated by my foolish attempt to learn in two weeks that which I had ignored for a lifetime. And since he was only beginning to learn about lymphoma, he could not possibly be the expert he thought I expected him to be. He had also begun to comprehend the severity of the disease, suspected that I didn't, and feared that any explanation he might give could possibly dampen my enthusiasm or lower my spirits—which he still saw as cheerful and positive, despite my unrealistic expectation of becoming an expert scientist overnight.

During that time before our next visit with Dr. Kaminski, I wanted to spend as much time as possible attempting to understand what my own body was trying to do to me. Although part of me wanted to maintain a normal work schedule, I quickly began to resent any interruption from my studies. I had work to do to save my own neck.

When I met with one of our clients to help them choose paint color, my own impatience surprised even me. I had always enjoyed every phase of helping families plan and build their homes, but after two hours of agonizing between two shades of off-white, my patience turned to agitation. Didn't they know they were keeping me from something far more important than their stupid paint? Not only that, I wanted to scream at them, "It won't matter two months from now. Why don't you go home and spend time with your kids?" Didn't they know that two hours choosing between shades of off-white paint was robbing them of quality time with their family? Just what did they think was important, anyway? For me, life's priorities were coming into focus.

As we continued our lymphoma education, Alex and I also began to learn that Dr. Kaminski was one of the leading lymphoma experts in the country. Still, we hoped that his diagnosis was absolutely wrong. At least I still hoped. Alex would later tell me that he had almost given up all hope for an incorrect diagnosis and had begun to worry about the possibility of human error as we progressed through treatments. Wrong medications or incorrect interpretations could spell big trouble. I hadn't even considered that possibility.

Alex and I talked briefly about getting a second opinion. "People go to U of M for second opinions," Alex said, "but we'll do whatever we have to do. Check it out."

Before I could check anything out, a friend in another state asked if she could show my biopsy report to the pathologist at the hospital where she worked. Alex and I thought that would be an easy way to obtain a second opinion, so I faxed the report to her. Within hours, my friend sent a message stating that her pathologist did not believe that lymphoma was circulating in my bloodstream.

Alex and I were confused. Had we misunderstood

Dr. Kaminski? He had said that lymphoma was circulating in my bloodstream, hadn't he? I sent Judy a quick email and she confirmed what we thought we had heard. These two differing opinions were disconcerting, and we wrestled with whom to believe.

I called the National Cancer Institute and the Lymphoma Research Foundation and the American Cancer Society. Did I know that people from all over the world travel to the University of Michigan for second opinions? Alex had mentioned that. There were other clinics and physicians, of course, but did I realize how fortunate I was to live in Ann Arbor and not have to travel? Hmm. I hadn't given any thought to that. Did I know that Dr. Mark Kaminski was one of the world's leading experts in lymphoma? Well, his name had certainly appeared in enough articles for us to reach that conclusion. And did I know that U of M was one of a handful of hospitals designated by the National Cancer Institute as a Comprehensive Cancer Center? No, I didn't know that.

I learned that stringent criteria must be met in order to receive NCI's designation. Hospitals can call themselves a Comprehensive Cancer Center, but names can be deceiving. At NCI-designated centers, diverse scientific disciplines collaboratively address cancer issues that a single investigator could not solve alone. Scientists at these institutions are linked to one another as well as to patients. Together, in this multi-institutional setting, they conduct research and provide patients with the most advanced therapies.

Alex and I quickly concluded that we would place all

our trust in the people at U of M. We had just learned about the team approach at the clinic. Up until then, we had not realized that other doctors reviewed my case with Dr. Kaminski. Nor had we realized that the clinic's pathologists specialize in hematology cases. Meeting every Thursday, this team of specialists *was* my second opinion. In fact, there were twenty or so opinions in those meetings. It seemed not only logical to trust the people who study lymphoma—and only lymphoma—on a daily basis, but it also gave us a tremendous level of comfort.

We never doubted the competency of Dr. Kaminski or his team. Our only desire for a second opinion stemmed from the hope that we could find one to refute the diagnosis so that our lives could return to normal. And normal was all we really wanted. But that was not to be. The Invisible Invader had other plans for us.

Having finally accepted the disease and U of M, I peered ahead and sensed that we were entering into a long-term *relationship* with Dr. Kaminski and his colleagues, one, I supposed, that would be unlike any other I had ever had. What in the world were its terms? And exactly what did I really know about these people to whom I was entrusting my life? Besides the fact that their credentials were among the best, not much. And so we turned to our personal experiences to fill in the blanks.

We'd built enough homes for physicians to know that they represented a cross-section of personality types. Some were funny, others were serious. All had to be highly motivated and fiercely competitive to have been accepted into medical school, much less to have completed it. Yes, we'd occasionally seen that competitive spirit appear as arrogance, but thankfully, we'd never seen that trait in anyone at the clinic. Arrogance would not only have failed to win my trust, but it would have also intensified the emotional trauma that cancer inflicts.

Personally, we also knew many health care professionals who were driven by sheer dedication to their patients, to finding cures for diseases, and to teaching the next generation. Unless you happen to be a masochist, their schedules were not ones to envy. Meetings with our doctor clients were often rescheduled at the last minute or interrupted by pagers calling them back to the hospital or at least to the nearest phone. They weren't always home to help their kids with homework or to cheer them on at basketball games. We'd witnessed missed birthdays, missed soccer games, missed piano recitals. We'd seen many health care professionals do all this and much more, always quietly and unpretentiously, in order to help others. And now those others included me, and I wished that I could somehow express my gratitude to those dedicated people and to their families who make enormous sacrifices.

And so, as I reflected on the physician/patient relationship ahead of me, I chose to draw from the best examples of health care professionals we had personally known to remind me that many are truly committed to their work. Even if my professional contact with previous doctors had made me feel that I was buying impersonal, "off the rack" medicine, Dr. Kaminski and Judy had so far made me feel that I had entered some sort of exclusive medical boutique. They had nearly dispelled my fear of an impersonal health care system by taking the time to learn my name, not just my patient number, and by patiently answering all our questions, which I tried to limit to a reasonable number, without ever making us feel dumb for not knowing the answers. They had even answered questions we had not known to ask.

It also seemed that Dr. Kaminski was not only an expert in lymphoma, but he and his colleagues were also beginning to convince me that they were experts in protecting the human spirit. He and Judy had tried to assure us that many people can live normal lives with lymphoma, and they had warned us that fear diminishes the quality of life for others. They had encouraged us to live our normal lives, and to think of myself as well while they worked to increase the length and quality of my life. Intuitively knowing that we were wrestling with uncertainties, they offered assurances and cheerfulness in generous proportions, and I grew confident that they were as devoted to their work as any of the best models I had ever seen. And because they were treating me as a real human being, it seemed only fair to extend the same courtesy.

But how? Besides simply trying to be pleasant, it also seemed that my expectations should be realistic. Again I turned to years of observing people in our own business, and I remembered that the clients who worked *with* us through the building process had a much easier and happier experience than the ones who placed impossible demands on us. I recalled a client some years back who had wanted us to remove a structural column in the basement in order to accommodate his furniture arrangement. Never mind that its placement had been carefully engineered to support the first and second floors, or that the building inspectors would never have approved the structure had we done so. The buyer refused to accept the necessity of that column, much less the ramifications of its removal, and neither his money nor his screaming and whining could make us remove it. Yes, experience told me that I'd be a whole lot happier in my unhappy situation if I worked *with* Dr. Kaminski. Still unsure exactly how, at least I figured out that I would set myself up for disappointment if I placed unrealistic expectations on him. Even the best doctors can't always put scrambled eggs back in the shell, but I was quite confident that Dr. Kaminski would do his best.

By the time Alex and I met with him and Judy on March 11, I had succeeded in putting a tremendous amount of pressure on myself, but had failed to cram medical school into two weeks. At least I had learned a few facts, and I thought I was ready to hear whatever Dr. Kaminski had to say. I wasn't.

It was time, he said, to begin treatment. I'd known that my counts were rising because Judy had been faithfully reporting the results of the blood tests since we'd last met. But hold on, Dr. Kaminski, I just figured out what a cell is. Let's not get ahead of me. With his usual patience and diplomacy, he recited our options and asked what we wanted to do. What did we want to do? We simply wanted to get rid of the Invisible Invader. Period. Rewind life and start the year over without lymphoma. And how was I supposed to choose one of the options? I hadn't finished medical school yet.

All I could think about was undergoing chemotherapy only to have the disease recur. The best we could hope for was to send it into remission for awhile, which in plain English translates to a temporary stay of execution. Wasn't there any way to get rid of it? Unfortunately not.

Dr. Kaminski repeated the hefty arsenal of treatments he had explained at our first meeting, and he again told us that it was best to start with the light artillery and work our way up to the big guns. I wanted to be glad that Dr. Kaminski had so many weapons, but I recoiled at the thought of every one of them.

I'll be forever grateful to Dr. Kaminski for the patience with which he repeated the pros and cons of each of the various treatments. I listened as carefully as I could while my mind raced through all the possibilities. Still, I was unable to make a decision. I turned to Alex to make it for me, but his expression indicated that he was as confused and overwhelmed as I. I told Dr. Kaminski that I simply did not know how to make this decision. What, Alex and I asked, would he do if I were his wife or daughter?

Dr. Kaminski recommended a clinical trial during which a chemotherapy called CVP would be administered eight times, once every three weeks. If I stayed in remission for six months after the chemotherapy, I would have a two-to-one chance of receiving a vaccine to fight the cancer.

Alex and I had read about these trials during the previous two weeks, but I was not ready to commit. Although I had resolved to be strong, I felt little strength then. I think I wanted Alex to decide for me. I certainly didn't feel competent to make the most important decision I had ever made in my life. And my fear of chemo made me want to buy at least a few days. It was Monday. We asked Dr. Kaminski if we could let him know by Thursday. He agreed.

We had scheduled meetings with clients on Monday and Tuesday nights. That left Wednesday night to review our options. Just as Alex and I began, Zan walked into the room and announced that he needed to get some schoolwork he had left at his mother's house. She had company and couldn't possibly bring it to him. Stunned, I thought, "She has *what*? We're trying to figure out how to save my life." Alex drove Zan to retrieve his papers while I sat home and fumed. Balancing a normal life with major decisions and medical treatment was going to require some effort.

Alex returned within a half-hour and we re-read the information about the clinical trial as well as about the other treatments Dr. Kaminski had explained. We talked about the options, but only briefly. I think we were already so tired of it all that we quickly agreed that the vaccine offered the most promise and hope at the moment.

On Friday, we were to meet with one of Dr. Kaminski's colleagues, Dr. Andrej Jakubowiak, to learn more about the clinical trial. I still wanted to know as much about lymphoma as the doctors knew, and I was frantically holding on to a faint hope that they were wrong. On the way to our appointment, I meekly asked Alex if he thought there was any possibility of a mistake. My heart sank as he answered that he thought the chances were slim.

In the examining room, Marian Blaesser, Dr. Jakubowiak's nurse practitioner, examined me. Much to my surprise, she had hardly entered the room when Alex asked what the chances were that all these test results were wrong. Marian must have heard that question before because she patiently explained the odds. None. Too many tests had confirmed the same thing. Alex had tried, and I loved him for his effort.

Marian sensed my frustration about not fully understanding lymphoma. She answered several questions until Dr. Jakubowiak arrived, and he answered many more. Still, it wasn't enough. Recognizing my apprehension, Marian told me the same thing that Dr. Kaminski and Judy had tried to tell me, but which I had not heard because I had first denied the disease and then attempted to learn too much too fast. She simply stated, "Betsy, it takes many years to learn about lymphoma, and even then, we don't always understand everything about it. The best thing you can do is let us understand it for you while you keep yourself strong."

In the frenzy I had been in, it would have been easy to take Marian's comment as condescending, but the compassion in her voice told me she was sincerely trying to help me. And at that moment, I quit medical school. After all, I had a whole team of some of the best doctors in the country to worry about the technical details of my disease and to help me fight it. My role became very clear. I would follow every instruction, report any change, answer all questions thoroughly, and otherwise keep myself as healthy and as positive as I could. Marian had lifted one enormous weight off my shoulders.

I signed the necessary papers for the clinical trial. Another CT scan and a bone marrow biopsy would be necessary in order for me to qualify for the clinical trial. Qualify? Gee, couldn't I try out for something more fun and less painful? How about a patient pin-up calendar?

Throughout the appointment, Alex sat in the chair while I sat on the examining table. His normal poker face had remained in the parking lot that morning. There was that mask of fear I had seen once before, and it tore at my heart. As Marian and I went to the front desk to make the necessary appointments, my eyes filled with tears for Alex. I'll never forget Marian putting her arm around my shoulder, trying to comfort me. "I've never met that man before today. He's in such pain," she said.

"I know, and I don't know how to make him feel better," I lamented. Alex would later tell me that on that day, he realized that the Invisible Invader was not going to leave as quickly as we had hoped. He hated the thought of my undergoing chemotherapy. And he was just beginning to grasp that head cheerleader was going to be a very difficult role.

CHAPTER FIVE

ROCKY

I'm sure that my maiden name—Kurka—predisposed me to cowardice. In Polish, "kurka" means "little chicken," and the only more appropriate name would have been whatever word means "big chicken," which is what I had always been when it came to needles, the sight of blood, and anything gory. So far I had somehow managed to tolerate all the blood tests with unusual aplomb, although I always turned my head away during the poke. When it came to anything that had to do with blood or guts, I didn't want to see it, hear about it, or talk about it.

During my short stint in medical school, I'd read that a bone marrow biopsy was a pretty uncomfortable procedure. A needle, three-sixteenths of an inch in diameter, would be inserted into the bone marrow and then attached to a syringe which would draw out the marrow. Regardless of how well I thought I had done so far, I really dreaded this procedure. I could just see a jackhammer tearing through my bone, followed by Roto Rooter s-l-u-r-p-ing out sludge through a vacuum hose. *And* I had the whole weekend to fret about it.

When Juli and I spoke on Saturday, she asked if I had been told what to expect. Yes, and I was less than thrilled. Did they tell you they would medicate you? No, I was to be awake during the procedure. "Mom, you really don't want to do that." No kidding. A nurse herself, Juli suggested, "We give our patients a drug called Versed. They're awake but remember nothing," she said. "Don't be afraid to ask for that or something like it. You may have to have another bone marrow biopsy sometime, and it will be much easier if you don't dread it."

Fully aware of my aversion to needles and such, Juli asked if anyone had told me about a port. A port? No, but I needed a port during this storm. How about one in the Bahamas? She explained that cancer patients require many procedures, including frequent blood draws. And chemotherapy can make the veins tired and tender. She went on to say that we had one good thing going for us, and that was our "great" veins. "Thanks, Mom," she said, "for the ugly hands you gave me. Our veins are everywhere, but in your case, they are going to be helpful to you."

But what about this port she was talking about? I'd read a little about ports, and Juli further explained that they were small objects surgically placed beneath the skin through which all needles for blood draws and infusions could be inserted. Disgusting. "I couldn't imagine looking at something like that," I said, "much less feeling it."

"Well," Juli suggested, "you might want to ask your doctor what he thinks about it. It might make your life a lot easier." I guess Dr. Kaminski thought I had great veins, too, because I never did get a port.

For the first time, I saw Juli's nursing skills in action, and I was very proud of her. My daughter, all grown-up with babies of her own, was lending a caring hand to me when I needed it most. I was just beginning to grasp the vital role nurses play in patient care.

The big day for my clinical trial tryout came. March 18. Should I wear something special? Do my nails? Draw smiley faces on my hips? Early on, I had resolved to muster as much dignity as I possibly could during whatever procedures the doctors ordered. I didn't want anyone to know what a chicken I really was, and I certainly didn't want to whine too much to the people who were trying to help me. But I was nervous about this bone marrow biopsy, and I hoped that I could maintain a brave face, despite the fact that I was convinced I would suffer great pain.

Carolyn Shearer, the physician's assistant who would do the procedure, came in to explain what she was going to do and how I would feel. It wouldn't take long, she assured me. Great, just a few minutes of agony and I could go home with my sore keister and painful memories. She could go home to whatever she went home to and sit comfortably. Lucky Carolyn. Poor me.

Carolyn was waiting to begin jackhammering when Dr. Craig Okada, principal investigator of this trial, arrived to draw the blood which would determine whether it was adequate to make the vaccine. Dr. Okada talked more about the trial and about lymphoma, and then he turned to Carolyn and asked when I was going to get medicated. I wasn't, she answered, as I sat on the table with this jingle rattling in my head:

> *I'll lie upon my tummy. My back will face the ceiling.*
> *Oh, good Lord, I'm really scared of what*
> *I'll soon be feeling.*
> *I'll pull my pants down to my thighs.*
> *I'll moon all in the room*
> *While Carolyn roots around my buns*
> *for marrow to exhume.*
> *She said I'd feel some pressure.*
> *Had she ever had this done?*
> *Was excruciating pain to be inflicted on each bun?*
> *She'll probably don a hardhat,*
> *put jackhammer in her hand.*
> *I hope I'll pass out quickly.*
> *Now wouldn't that be grand?*
> *Bandaged up, she'll send me home*
> *with my sore derriere.*
> *Oh, I pray with all my heart bad lymphocytes*
> *aren't there.*

Dr. Okada became my new best friend that day. He thought it would be a good idea to give me some Versed so that I could be more comfortable through the procedure. There was some discussion about when I had last eaten, and it was decided that the procedure would have to be postponed for two hours if I wanted the Versed. Wanted it?

Bring it on! I botched everyone's schedules that day, but I wanted to throw my arms around Dr. Okada's neck. Not only had he prescribed the drug, but he'd also spared me the embarrassment of begging for it!

Thanks to Versed, I really don't remember anything about the first bone marrow biopsy. Alex returned after the procedure, gave me a big hug, and took me home by late afternoon.

Two days later I flew to Virginia to visit my mother and sister. For the past few years, Mother, at ninety-two, had divided her time between our house and Karen's, but her congestive heart failure was worsening and she was traveling less frequently to visit us. Though her heart leaked like a sieve, she refused surgery to correct it, and the doctors felt that her chances of surviving surgery were slim anyway. For the past five or six years, she had landed in the hospital two or three times each year. Her blood pressure would read 250-ish over 11 or 12, and the doctors would shake their heads in amazement that she survived these bouts, but she would always wake up with a smile and say, "Well, I'm still here."

Still, I knew she would not live forever. Once I started chemo, I feared that travel might be difficult, and I wanted to visit her as soon as possible. Karen and I had deliberated about whether to tell her what was happening to me. Mother's comprehension and memory had diminished in recent years, and we did not want to worry her. After all, she had already lost one child, and we didn't want her to worry about losing another. On the other hand, we agreed that we owed her a certain amount of honesty. We decided to tell her very briefly without actually saying "cancer," a word her generation considered a death sentence.

I gave considerable thought to how I would break this news to Mother. I knew that her optimistic nature would be helpful to all of us, and I smiled at the thought of her as a person, not just as my mother. She is one of the most gracious ladies you could ever hope to meet. She's a true Southern belle, the daughter of prim Victorian parents from whom she inherited her deep-seated beliefs of what was and wasn't proper for young ladies, old ladies, and every lady in between. Among other things, she taught me to wear white shoes only between Memorial Day and Labor Day, and only to wear white shoes if you positively could not find shoes to match your outfit. Women were not supposed to work, but to marry young and have babies just as she and my sisters had done. It was her idea of what was proper.

For years I had judged my mother as a rigid product of an irrelevant era, and I had resented it. Why had she influenced me to marry young instead of recognizing that women were changing and taking their place in the world? By the time I was in my late thirties, I had come to realize that my mother had raised me within the only frame of reference she knew, and I realized how much I had learned from her, including the power to think positively. She had taught me, by example, that little acts of kindness could brighten the days of others. And what was the use of complaining? It only made those around you miserable. "Look around," she would say, "when you think you have no shoes. You'll always find someone else who has no feet."

Lymphoma would make me admire my mother's attitude more than ever before. Her wisdom would give me strength. And, even at my age, re-examining her and my father's influences—the ones that had shaped me—helped to build a foundation under my insecurities.

During the first evening of my visit, over dinner, I explained to Mother that I had a blood disorder. My white blood cells weren't dying after they divided, and too many cells could be harmful. Immediately, she asked if having me late in her life had caused this. I felt so sorry that she might blame herself, and I assured her she had nothing to do with it. Doctors didn't know what caused it, but they could fix it. "How?" she wanted to know. They'd put me on some strong medicine over the course of about six months. I'd probably lose my hair and may not be able to travel to see her, but I would otherwise feel fine.

Mother never asked if I had cancer or if the treatment I was describing was chemo. I'm not sure if she simply didn't want to know or didn't think to inquire. She was, however, very concerned about me, and I assured her that I would be fine. I joked that if my cells lived indefinitely, then surely so would I.

Our conversation was over almost as quickly as it had begun. Mother understood that I was sick, but it ended there. Mentally, she was too frail to sit through the details of some strange disease and too frail for me to lean on for strength.

Still, I felt safe and peaceful sitting across from her at the dinner table at Karen's house. Far from home, the Invisible Invader felt distant, as if it had stayed behind in Michigan. When my visit came to an end four days later, it was hard to make myself get on the plane and return to the disease and to the chemotherapy that was waiting for me. Much worse, I wondered what I would do if Mother went into the hospital—or died—and I was too sick to travel. As we said goodbye at the airport, I couldn't help but wonder if this would be the last time I would see her. I prayed that it would not be.

I had also wanted to squeeze in a quick trip to Florida to see Juli and the babies. Although I saw them every two to three months, I'd always wished I could live two lives— one in Michigan and one in Florida—and now more than ever I desperately needed to see them. But since schools were on spring break, all flights were overbooked on the only days I could go. Those planes were loaded with families and college students headed for fun in the sun while I was headed straight for chemo. I was frantic about when I would see Juli and my grandchildren again.

The day after returning from Virginia, I drove to the hospital for another CT scan. Two weeks to go before starting chemo. During that time, the blood tests and bone marrow biopsy indicated that I had made the cut for the vaccine tryouts. I was absolutely positive that I would be selected to receive the magic vaccine, after which all would be fine and life could return to normal. Always realistic, Alex accepted the two-to-one odds better than I.

During those two weeks, I worked maniacally, afraid of when I might be able to work again. And I tried to psych myself up for chemo. Actually, I tried to psych myself up for learning how to maintain dignity while throwing up in front of other people. I could hardly wait.

Juli had sent me a book entitled *Getting Well Again* by O. Carl Simonton, Stephanie Matthews-Simonton, and James L. Creighton. I had read it cover to cover and had started to practice the guided imagery the book teaches. Self-training became a daily exercise, although it wasn't much different than what I had done for years. At work, for example, I'd never called it guided imagery, but I'd always used the empowerment of positive images to guide me. For example, I always envisioned writing a contract when I met with a prospective client. What I had to do now was use my imagination to visualize the cancer cells leaving my body. I'm not certain that I practiced it exactly according to the book, but my version of guided imagery did become a tool that calmed me, made the treatments more bearable, and helped me to expect success.

I also attended my first lymphoma support group meeting. Held at the hospital, it was co-facilitated by Judy and Claudia Ouimet-Dillon, a social worker specializing in cancer. Alex had no interest in going. Frankly, I was drawn more by morbid curiosity than a need to find support. Who would be there? What would they look like? Would they appear ill and maybe even deformed by the disease or medical procedures? How did they feel? I needed to know.

Much to my relief, everyone looked healthy and normal. Some had completed various treatments and had been in remission for some time. One had begun treatment recently.

Others were still watching and waiting. All of us were hopeful.

The woman who had recently begun treatment was about my age. She told us that for several years she'd had hot flashes and an enlarged lymph node on her leg which was dismissed as insignificant. Her previous gynecologist had diagnosed her as menopausal, and had even scheduled her for a hysterectomy when another doctor had ordered a blood test and—*voilà!*—found lymphoma.

I sat there listening to this woman's story wondering what medical schools teach in Hot Flashes 101, and I thought that it was time to rewrite the syllabus for that course so that every single known cause for hot flashes, including menopause and lymphoma, was taught. Looking beyond gynecological reasons may, in fact, save a life.

Dr. Joseph Himle, clinical assistant professor of psychology, spoke to the group that night. Alex had built a home for the Himles before I moved to Michigan, and together we had recently finished building another. Through building his family's home, I had gotten to know Joe as a delightful man with a wicked sense of humor. I'd never had the occasion to observe him professionally, and I wondered if I could sit in the same room with him without laughing.

It turned out that I could, although Joe interjected some humor into his talk where it was appropriate. He described depression as a common side effect of cancer, explained how to recognize it, and offered some advice to combat it. One of his ideas had a strong impact on me. As an example of how powerful our minds can be, he proposed that if each of us were to write on a three-by-five card the five things about which we felt most guilty in our lives, and we were to look at that card every hour for a day, we'd probably end up feeling pretty badly. Couldn't we also make ourselves feel better by reminding ourselves of positive things?

At home that night, I found a three-by-five card. I reasoned that I could at least manage my mental health even if I couldn't control my physical ailment, and so I wrote across the top of the card, "If you can worry yourself sick, you can think yourself well." I realized that I had far more blessings than would fit on the card. I wrote the ones that would give me the most hope—Alex, Juli, Skye, Nicholas, and the other family and friends I treasured most. I tucked the card away just in case I might need it, and I knew whom I'd be calling if I even thought that my mental state was collapsing. By the end of the summer, that card would be well-worn as I struggled to find beacons of hope.

The Lymphoma Research Foundation has a wonderful peer support program which matches patients to others who have been in similar situations. They put me in touch with a gentleman in California who had gone through the same clinical trial, and our conversation was very helpful. He assured me he had been able to continue working during most of the chemo treatment. Yes, there were days he was tired. Yes, he sometimes felt jittery while taking the prednisone. He had also had some constipation throughout. Great, here I was talking about constipation with a total stranger. How weird was that? He also told me that he believed yoga, guided imagery, and a good diet had helped him cope. Our conversation left me feeling that this wouldn't be so bad. I could do it. No problem.

During those last two weeks before chemo began, I was Rocky getting ready for the fight. No doubt about it. By the weekend before it started, I was ready. At least that's what I wanted everyone else to think. It was all an act. I hated my body for its attack on me, and I wanted nothing to do with any of this. But I kept telling myself that if chemo and the vaccine could save my life, then I would tolerate any unpleasant side effects.

Alex, too, was clearly bewildered by the situation we faced. When I asked him how he was doing, he tried to assure me that he was fine, but the sadness in his eyes was unconvincing. I told him that it was okay to be sad or angry or disappointed, and I often encouraged him to share his feelings, but he would just put his arms around me and tell me not to worry about him. How could I *not*? I desperately wanted to alleviate his pain, but he remained stoic and unwilling, or perhaps unable, to verbalize his private agony, for which I felt responsible. I thus felt that I must play his comforter, and yet I could find nothing with which to comfort him.

I believed then, as I do now, that patients' attitudes have a significant effect on how our families and friends react to our illnesses. Consequently, it was my responsibility to create an atmosphere of hope for Alex and others who cared about me, a conviction I tried to sustain, but which sometimes languished under the weight of my own subsequent fears and doubts. But at that time, I yearned for ways to lighten the melodrama so that those around me would find some consolation. Knowing little else to do, I turned to humor, however feeble, to provide temporary relief. My hair dryer and curling iron would take a vacation, and I was sure we'd save at least fifty cents on the electric bill. Spring was coming, so our cat and I would bond in the spring shedding ritual. On and on I went. Whenever and however I could, I tried to crack jokes to make everyone around me laugh, believing that was what people expected of me. But mostly, the jokes were my way of saying, "Everything will be okay." Unfortunately, Alex was never amused by anything I said or did, but there is no doubt that he would have fared worse had I been morose.

I made an appointment to have my hair cut the day after chemo started. That was a big step. When I was seven years old, my mother had cut my hair short and given me a home perm. I had thought I looked like a freak, and I think it scarred me for life. I vowed I would never have short hair again, and I didn't. In my late forties, I did shorten it up to my shoulders, but it had never been much shorter than that. Making the appointment to have it whacked off was a big step, but giving up some of my hair, on my own terms, gave me some sense of control over my life and over how much mess I would make when I started to shed.

Resentful that I had to spend money on something I did not even want, I shopped for a wig at a medical supply store. The saleswoman directed me to a room full of wigs and closed the door so that I could have some privacy. I hated every one I tried on. They looked and felt awful. She never told me they could be trimmed or styled. I left, wigless, in tears.

How much time did I have before my hair would fall out? Who knew? Everyone is different. Since summer was coming, I decided I'd wear fun, fashionable hats, so I headed to the mall and tried on every one in every store. Have you ever tried to find fashionable hats that actually cover every part of a denuded cranium? There are few, and I cursed the milliners for designing perky little fashion statements for only the healthy. Maybe none of them had ever had cancer. I finally found a couple, although I can't say that I was pleased with my purchases.

I worried about how I would maintain our home, which we had recently put on the market with the intention of moving midsummer. Our move would make the new house our fifth home in seven years. Moving was simply a way of life. Not my way of life, necessarily, but Alex's.

I'd always teased Alex that most builders, if not all, must directly descend from nomads who, I theorized, wandered the countryside in search of the most desirable real estate. Despite generations of intermarriage, nomadic genes dominated in several bloodlines. The progeny would invariably become builders whose real purpose remains the same as their forefathers, which is, of course, to acquire the best real estate before someone else does. But without a universally accepted definition of "best," builders continue their quixotic search by frequently changing addresses—which is what we expected to do all too soon again, and I wasn't quite certain how I was supposed to manage it.

The evening before chemo began, Karen called to wish me luck. Always practical, she suggested I prepare a garbage can with a plastic bag so that I could neatly dispose of its contents. I'd thought in abstract terms about vomiting, but this suggestion put me ever closer to the actual reality.

Karen continued with another practical suggestion. In case I became sick on the way home, it would be a good idea to take a plastic bag in the car. Sick in the car on the way home? In front of Alex? Oh God, I hadn't thought about that. I'd estimated we would leave the hospital at rush hour, and I could just see myself spewing vomit as we waited for the light at the crowded intersection of Jackson and Maple. I'd throw up not only in front of Alex, but also in front of all the passengers in surrounding cars. I couldn't bear the thought. Even if chemo finished during daylight hours, surely we shouldn't leave the hospital until after dark. I was totally grossed out by the thought of throwing up, much less in the car, but reality was speeding at me. Just how was I going to maintain any dignity?

Juli also called that evening. When I confided my fears to her, she did her best to assure me that the anti-nausea drugs work pretty well, and she promised to send anti-nausea vibes all during the next day. I was so grateful for the pep talk my daughter gave me that night.

Still, Rocky wasn't really ready for the fight. Rocky had never wanted this fight in the first place. I went to bed trying to think positive thoughts and trying to practice guided imagery, but fear superseded every good thought. Naturally, I didn't want anyone to know that I had switched into full-blown panic mode.

Like me, Alex continued to conceal his real feelings, but he would much later reveal that he had been gearing up for this battle, too. Practically, he was working even harder to keep a sharp eye on all the balls he was juggling while trying to make certain that he never stumbled. Emotionally, fear of the unknown was emerging. While I seemed to worry mostly about the initial treatment, he tried to peer beyond it and to formulate a clear plan to help me through the coming months. But as he said later, "How can anyone plan without knowledge of what to plan for? And how could I plan to help without knowing what help you would need?"

At the time, Alex did not want to raise the subject of potential complications that I might not have considered, but he was fully aware that side effects vary widely and hoped that mine would be minimal. If they took a great physical toll, he worried that I might lose my will to fight and that he would not know how to motivate me to stay in the fray. Despite huge efforts to deny all but positive thoughts, those what-ifs he had vowed to suppress were beginning to penetrate his resolve.

CHAPTER SIX

DOPE-ON-A-ROPE

In my former life, the most I knew, or thought I knew, about chemotherapy was that it was a drug used in the treatment of cancer. As usual, I was only partly right. In reality, chemotherapy is a term for a group of chemicals. Used singly or in combination, they have a specific toxic effect on disease-producing organisms.

I was to receive a combination of cyclophosphamide, vincristene, and prednisone, which is commonly called CVP. Cyclophosphamide is one of the group of alkylating agents which disrupts many normal functions of DNA, including its ability to divide. Vincristine is a tubulin-binding agent which also stops the cell from dividing. Prednisone, an immune suppressant, suppresses the rampant growth of cancerous white blood cells. The "C" and "V" components would be injected, while I would take the prednisone in pill form for five days thereafter. In plain English, the chemo would commit cellular genocide and grant me a stay of execution.

That was all good. It was the quality of life during and after chemo that didn't sound exactly rosy. During my brief but accelerated stint in medical school, I had reviewed the list of potential side effects of various drug combinations, and I had learned that chemotherapy could imperil my veins, my heart, my liver, my lungs, and just about every other organ in my body. A partial list of collateral damage could include mouth sores, hair loss, fatigue, insomnia, weight gain, weight loss, gastric ulcers, diabetes, cataracts, glaucoma, high blood pressure, blood clots, constipation, diarrhea, seizures, rapid mood changes from euphoria to depression, and, occasionally, psychosis.

See the problem? Even the medicine couldn't make up its mind whether to give me diarrhea or constipation, insomnia or fatigue, weight gain or weight loss, euphoria or depression. *And*, in exchange for one affliction, I could end up with several. Who wouldn't be psychotic?

On April 8, I awoke bargaining with God, as I had so often done in previous weeks. If You want me to undergo this chemotherapy, would You please help the chemicals do their job? And one more thing. If it's not too much to ask, could You please keep the side effects to a bare minimum? I really *did* want to live. And be healthy enough to enjoy life.

I climbed out of bed, went downstairs for coffee and oatmeal, and returned upstairs to prepare myself for my own voluntary metamorphosis into a toxic waste dump. Standing in the closet, I wondered what was appropriate attire for such an occasion. Perhaps something complementary to my own vomit in case it became an unwanted accessory later? Comfort reigned supreme, and I chose an old black pantsuit. Black seemed appropriate. I was, after all, mourning my good health.

As I prepared myself that morning, I examined—really examined—myself in the mirror, something I had never spent much time doing. I'd never counted wrinkles or bothered with facials. I didn't slop on night creams or morning creams, and hadn't searched for flaws to cover. But that morning, I scrutinized my face, and for the first time, beheld the imperfections and faults and furrows the world saw on my fifty-one-year-old face. None of them troubled me. They were simply natural affirmations of living life for just over half a century, but I shuddered at the thought that the drugs or the disease might accelerate the natural aging process. How long before a shriveled stranger would peer back from the mirror? I tried to commit my face to memory, just as it was that morning.

Enroute to the hospital by eight AM, Alex and I chattered about work, but we both knew it was a feeble attempt to avoid thinking about the inevitable, now just moments away. I wondered where people in all the surrounding cars were going. To work? To school? To the gym? Weren't they the lucky ones? Couldn't we just turn around and start the day over? Do something different?

Digressing from our idle conversation, I asked Alex how he was feeling. "This all seems so surreal," he said. "An out-of-body experience." Funny, that's exactly what I was thinking. Like an episode from *The Twilight Zone*, we were looking down at our other selves going to a place we would never voluntarily go.

For the next several minutes, we were silent. Then, at

the traffic light where we would turn into the hospital complex, Alex turned to face me and added that he felt so out of control, so helpless. I'd known that. Men are fixers. When something breaks, they simply go to the hardware store, buy the necessary part, bring it home, and fix it. And when they can't do that, they feel out of control. I joked that we should run by Stadium Hardware and see if they had some Super-Duper Immune Fixative. Without laughing, he said, "I wish."

In the parking lot, Alex shut off the ignition, turned to me again, and sighed. I shifted to face him, smiled, and sighed back. "Okay. How about this? We'll just drop my body off at Dr. Kaminski's Body Repair, you and I will hop a plane for the Caribbean, and we'll pick it up when he's done. What do you think?"

Ignoring my absurdity, he said, "I hate that you have to do this."

"It's not my idea of fun either, but let's go and get it over with." We hugged and walked hand in hand to the clinic.

In the waiting room, Alex leaned over and placed his elbows on his knees and his forehead in the palms of his hands. I rubbed his back and asked what he was thinking. Slowly, he lowered one hand. Still cradling his head in the other, he turned to look up at me. Did I see a little tear in one eye? He sheepishly grinned and answered, "I think I need a drink."

"Have one for me," I told him.

We met with Dr. Kaminski and Judy in the examining room where they inspected me one final time before chemo.

They asked if we had any more questions, but we were too numb to think of any. Both wished us well and assured us they would be nearby if we needed them.

When we checked in at the infusion desk, the receptionist gave me a message from Juli. It said, "Remember the vibes I'm sending you today. Good luck. I love you." My eyes dampened, and I clutched that note for a very long time that day.

The Lymphoma Clinic and the infusion area share a reception area, so I had been there before. But suddenly, I wondered if everyone would be tossing their cookies. Would the whole place reek? I almost gagged just thinking about it.

I tried to keep my spirits up and think positively. This CVP was surely an acronym for a Cure is Very Promising. Silently, I repeated all the jokes I had cracked. I had even brought work to review with Alex—anything to take my mind off the pollutants that would soon enter my body. I was anxious to slay the Invisible Invader as soon as possible, but on the other hand, I was apprehensive about chemo's side effects. Apprehension was winning.

I had to go to the bathroom. Once I left Alex, my eyes filled with tears, and I stared straight down so that no one would see. Without looking, I pushed open the bathroom door and walked to the first stall. There I sat, tears and pee flowing in perfect sync. I hadn't heard the door open, but I suddenly realized that there was a strong flow going outside my stall. It didn't sound quite right. Then I heard the door open again. Footsteps. A man's voice. Another man's voice and another strong flow.

How was I going to get out of this predicament? Maybe I could just wait until they left and no one would be any wiser. I lifted my legs off the floor so they wouldn't see women's shoes. Couldn't they just finish and leave? Should I flush and flee? One man left, and I thought the other would be out of there soon and that I could make an escape unnoticed. But then another man came in. I'll never get out of here, I thought, not without being seen. Finally, I put my head down, opened the stall door and ran, mumbling, "Sorry," as I bolted through the door. I dashed to the couch where Alex was sitting and buried my head in his shoulder, whimpering, "I just went into the men's room."

"What did you do that for?" he asked. I explained that I put my head down on the way to the bathroom because I was about to cry and never looked at which door I opened. Shaking his head, he put his arm around me and tried to comfort me. I don't think Alex has ever made such a dumb mistake. Even in the worst crisis, he observes everything around him. Was I already losing my ability to function in a normal world? Would I need to have Alex walk me to a bathroom? And why couldn't they call my name now? How long would I have to sit in that waiting room with the men who had seen me dash out of the men's room?

I froze when my name finally was called. I remember looking at Alex and thinking that if I just didn't answer, we could silently escape down the elevator and forget about all this.

Looking back, I wish I had asked Dr. Kaminski or Judy

for a tour of the infusion area before chemo began. I would have seen that people were not throwing up. I would have seen that it was not the torture chamber I had envisioned.

Instead, the bright, semicircular room was lined with reclining chairs. Patients, some awake and some asleep, were attached to IVs. No one was sick and the room had no odor, thank goodness. An aide escorted us to my own recliner where I settled in with a mixture of trepidation and hope.

A nurse stopped by, made small talk about her children and her job, asked about mine, and otherwise did her best to assure me that I would be just fine. Another aide came and offered to bring us a bagel or juice. That was a surprise. I hadn't expected room service—or rather chairside service.

Alex sat facing me, clearly wondering what to expect. Silently, he was thinking that he wished this was all behind us. He wanted to remain optimistic and thought to himself, "This better work." But he had read enough to understand that no chemo comes with a guarantee. Since I had never expressed that concern, he certainly didn't want to raise that unhappy possibility, and he tried to banish the thought from his mind in order to hide his worry from me. But there was no hiding his worry. The anguish in his eyes clearly told me how difficult it was for him to watch a stranger pump my body full of lethal chemicals.

There was no escape now, for him or for me, so I surrendered to the inescapable. I winced as the nurse inserted the IV and hung the bag of chemicals. With a smile, I gave Alex the thumbs up sign, pointed to the drugs hanging high above my shoulder, fondled the tube through which they dripped, and declared with conviction, "This Dope-On-A-Rope gives me lots of hope." Indeed, that bag was the SWAT team sent to massacre a vulnerable enemy. At least I hoped it was vulnerable.

Within minutes, my eyelids became too heavy to lift, and my mind drifted to images of myself as a gray-haired old lady walking hand in hand with Alex on a beach. Warm, foamy waves gently lapped at our feet while seagulls cried overhead. That's the last thing I remember before I fell asleep.

I neither threw up nor saw anyone who did. I was groggy when we left the hospital, but relieved that nothing horrible had happened. I didn't even feel nauseated. And when I awoke the next morning, I was surprised that I felt no different than I had the previous morning. How anticlimactic can you get?

Alex called as I was leaving for my hair appointment. "I've decided to shave my head in solidarity," he proudly proclaimed.

"Thanks," I laughed, "but don't even think about it."

"I'll do it," he repeated.

"No way," I insisted. He didn't, thank goodness. I would have felt badly had he taken that extra step because I knew how sensitive he was about his thinning hair. Anyway, he was supporting me in a myriad of other, more useful ways.

As my hairdresser began to cut my tresses, golden with assistance, I nervously awaited the outcome of this voluntary shearing. Within minutes, several inches of frosted locks lay discarded on the floor, revealing my natural color for the first time in many years. For the second day in a row, I stared at the image in the mirror, startled by the brown-haired lady with such short hair staring back. Was that really me?

Oddly enough, I disliked the cut less than the color. At least it wasn't gray, I mused. And most importantly, I had smugly preempted at least one aspect of the disease and established exactly who was in charge.

I don't know what Alex really thought, but when he first saw me with my new look, he smiled and said, "Hey, you look like Jamie Lee Curtis. Pretty chic." And as I encountered friends and acquaintances, they all told me how much younger I looked. Maybe I should have cut my hair years ago. It certainly reduced the time it took to get ready in the mornings.

I grew accustomed to the chemo cut in no time. Pregnancy had almost knocked out my eyebrows, so they were of little concern. I did wonder if my eyelashes would fall out. They didn't. I probably wouldn't have to shave my legs very often, I mused. And the best news was that those pesky little chin hairs that I was forever plucking wouldn't be a nuisance either. At least so I thought. In fact, those little chin hairs would mistake chemo for Miracle Gro, and they would multiply profusely. Go figure.

About five days after the first treatment, I realized that my intestines were painfully overloaded, another new experience for me. I drank an ocean of prune juice for two days before resorting to milk of magnesia. I suppose I expected the first dose to do the trick quickly, and when it didn't, I took more . . . and more. By the time the medicine bore its results, I joked about teaching United Van Lines a thing or two about moving.

Friends delivered mouthwatering dinners to us over the next few days and weeks. Because I was feeling perfectly fine, I was a little embarrassed about accepting their meals, delicious as they were. More deeply, I was humbled and self-conscious by the attention, especially from people whom I considered acquaintances. Cancer would require me to learn to accept help in many forms from many people. It would also teach me that family, friends, acquaintances, and even strangers welcomed the opportunity to participate in my healing.

Remembering my mother's wisdom, I decided to deflect the focus away from myself and to make a conscious effort to do more for others. I wrote notes to old friends. I sent funny cards for no reason at all. I baked cookies and cakes for the nurses who drew blood and administered the chemo, and for the doctors and their staffs who cared for me. I continued doing these things throughout my treatment, and it did help to lift my spirits. It wasn't until months later that I consciously realized that my efforts were not only a way of saying hello or thank you, but also a way of reminding people that I was still me, not just a blob of cancer.

During that first cycle of chemo, Alex and I were greatly relieved that none of our fears about side effects material-ized. I remained upbeat and thankful that I was able to continue to work and to lead a perfectly normal life, inter-rupted only by regular blood draws. Judy kept me well-informed that my counts were falling and rising as expected. When the time arrived for the second treatment, three weeks after the first, I was a seasoned chemo pro, and I waltzed into the infusion area, perfectly happy to have life-saving toxins enter my body.

By the second week of the second cycle, I was tiring more easily. I startled Alex one morning that week when he stopped by the house to retrieve a forgotten file and found me sound asleep with my head at the foot of the bed and my feet on the pillows. I'd gone upstairs to dress and found our cat Tooties curled at the foot of our bed. I curled up around him—just to give him a quick hug before showering—and fell sound asleep. It wasn't even nine in the morning.

Alex caught me snoozing again the following morning. I had spread blueprints out on the dining room table to make some changes to them. I don't remember putting my head down, but he found me sound asleep, sitting in the chair with my head on the blueprints. My naps were never long, but they were evidence of the drugs taking their toll.

My hair had not fallen out as I had expected. A strand or two stayed in the comb now and then, but Tooties was definitely winning the shedding race. I did pick up a wig, just in case I overtook my feline counterpart.

The third week of the second cycle began. I was exhausted, and on Monday morning, began to run a fever. Judy asked me to come to the clinic right away and suggested I plan for a hospital stay. This time, I called Alex and asked him to give me a ride.

CHAPTER SEVEN

HOTEL HELL

At the clinic, Judy and Dr. Kaminski determined that I had developed neutropenia, a side effect of chemotherapy resulting from the lowering of infection-fighting neutrophils. In plain English, my body was unable to fend off normal worldly germs, and they were was pestering me with some sort of microscopic blight. From the clinic, I was sent directly to a private cell in the hospital where I would have contact with no one except nurses and doctors. Large doses of antibiotics were pumped into me, and since other patients were out of sight, they were also out of mind. I still did not consider myself particularly ill, although I was. I was simply in some clinical hideaway for a small adjustment. It was an inconvenient but short incarceration of two days. Nothing more, nothing less.

However, one incident during my stay astounded me. Alex, sitting in the chair beside my bed, asked a nurse whether cancer could be contracted through bodily fluids. I sat straight up and stared at him in disbelief. There sat an intelligent man who had read about cancer and who should have known that he couldn't catch cancer from a kiss.

Months later I would learn that his fear was common, though unfounded. Cancer is not contagious. I guess Alex simply needed reassurance.

His other fears also surfaced. Although he hoped this would be our only complication, he had already realized that the road to recovery was going to be much harder than he had anticipated, and he searched himself for additional resolve with which to steel himself against further difficulties. Of course he did not share those thoughts with me at the time. He was too busy trying to wear his mask of optimism.

I was delighted to return home from the hospital, although I was exhausted. After just two days at home, however, another fever arose and a pain in my left midsection was increasing. By midday, when I literally crawled up the stairs on all fours, I reluctantly called Judy. I was afraid she would tell me to return to the clinic prepared for another hospital stay, which is exactly what she did.

I called Alex and asked him to put on his chauffeur's hat again. Within minutes, he was home to take me to the hospital for the second time that week. Just before leaving, I withdrew our home from the multiple listing service and removed the for sale sign from the yard. Somehow I knew it would be impossible to continue showing the house, at least for awhile. Packing, moving, and unpacking was inconceivable. Alex's nomadic wanderlust would have to wait.

It was a Friday afternoon when I was readmitted to the hospital. Alex and I rode the elevator to the eighth floor and disembarked to double doors announcing "Hematology

Oncology Unit/Bone Marrow Transplant/Restricted Area." Restricted from what? I'd never been on a floor in a hospital where double doors separated patients from the general hospital population. Those doors signified, in no uncertain terms, how sick Dr. Kaminski thought I was, and I choked up, wondering what was in store for me behind them. As he had so often done during this ordeal, Alex put his arms around me, imparting the necessary strength I needed to pass through the doors. Still, I felt like a repeat offender entering San Quentin. Worse, for the first time I saw myself for what I really was: a patient.

But just exactly what was a patient? If I had ever given any thought—which I hadn't—to the definition of "patient" in medical terms, I would have made some snide remark about doctors calling their clients "patients" because long waiting room waits required "patience." However, according to my dictionary, "patient" is a derivative of the Latin word "patiens" which means "to suffer." Given that root, I refused, mentally, to be one. I was happy to be a client, a consumer, a buyer, a purchaser, a customer, or even a loyal follower, but not a sufferer. And no, even if the moniker suggested I was actually purchasing medical services, I did not expect a buy-nine-visits-and-get-one-free card to arrive in the mail.

Unlike hospital floors where people recover from broken bones, it was clear that everyone on this floor suffered from a potentially fatal illness. Not to minimize broken bones, but it was very depressing to be thrust into the company of patients whose outcomes were possibly so final. As I looked around, however, it seemed that most were in worse condition than I, but were still receiving life-saving drugs. I convinced myself that if their doctors believed they had a chance, then surely mine was better. At least I had walked in on my own two feet.

I was escorted to a semi-private cell where I would be excluded from life for ten days. In case you don't know, semi-private is an oxymoron. There is nothing private about a hospital. Carts clang, bells ring, the PA system calls nurses and doctors at all hours of the day and night. Private bodily functions become public property. Sleep is permitted only between medications and tests, both of which are inflicted around the clock. Don't hospitals know that sleep deprivation has been a form of torture for centuries?

I scarcely settled into my room before a nurse thrust in an IV, to which I would be securely affixed for the duration of my visit. Complications everyone hopes to avoid went from bad to worse. If I had escaped feeling ill before, my reprieve was up. I felt horrible. The pain in my midsection was diagnosed as an infarct, or the death of part of my spleen. Just great, I thought. My body had decided I deserved a slow death and would kill me one part at a time. Then pneumonia set in. Worse, CVP wasn't doing its job. The headlines might have read, "The Invisible Invader Rolls Over Betsy, 1–0." When a stronger chemo was administered, renal failure followed, the result of tumor lysis syndrome which can arise when the contents of tumor cells are released as the cells are destroyed.

My first roommate, who arrived shortly after I did, was

an older lady whose husband never left her bedside, day or night. They kept the curtain between us drawn at all times and hardly spoke to each other, much less to me.

Alex, Lisa, Ted, Zan, and Greta visited throughout the weekend. Lisa, at eighty-four, hugged me and joked, "You better get well. I'm counting on you to take care of me." Without having any idea how I would deliver, I promised her that I would. Alex's face, blank and drawn, revealed his anxiety. He seemed remote, almost aloof. When I suggested he sit on the foot of the bed for lack of available chairs, he chose instead to stand. Although he said he was more comfortable standing—and, knowing Alex, he probably was—I interpreted his physical distance of a few feet as miles of emotional distance. Only when everyone was leaving did he approach, and then only long enough to give me a cursory kiss on the forehead.

Alex would later tell me that he had only thought he understood the seriousness of my illness before I landed in the hospital the second time. That weekend, he began to grasp its real danger as he watched me begin to spiral downward physically. Where I would stop was anyone's guess, and his own confidence and optimism plummeted with each new physical complication. Unable to sleep, he turned to Jack Daniels for assistance, but found little.

Alex also genuinely wanted to hide his fears from me, but even his stoicism made it difficult to manage a smile when he had no idea how far I would fall. Or how far he would. He resolved to be as encouraging to me as his remaining strength would allow, but he also feared that he would crumble if he came too close to me—and that was something he did not want me to see.

By Sunday evening, I felt wretched. I rarely dream, or at least don't remember dreams, but in the middle of that night, I had the most vivid dream I can ever remember. In full technicolor, I saw my father with his arms folded just as he had often held them. We were separated only by a narrow stream. He assured me, "Don't worry, everything is very comfortable where I am." I was sure Daddy was telling me that I would soon cross that stream and join him.

I awakened from this specter of death unnerved, terrified, and fighting for my life. Death had always been so abstract, but then it seemed so imminent, and I'd never felt so totally alone. I needed Alex, but I couldn't reach the phone. Instead, I called the nurse. Waiting for her, I wrote "Call Alex" on a notepad I could reach. I still have that note and now see how shaky my handwriting was.

No one called Alex in the middle of the night, and even now, I am not certain how much distress I was in. I remember very little about the following day, except that the dream haunted me. As much as I loved my father, I was hardly ready for a reunion.

Alex told me several months later that I had begged him that day not to keep me alive on life support. I reminded him that the hospital had a copy of my living will. Make sure they remember it, I demanded of him. I have no memory of that conversation, but Alex grew terrified that I was losing my will to fight the battle.

I do remember that oxygen was added to my daily

regimen. The tubes in my nose were reminders that I could no longer accomplish the small feat of breathing on my own. I felt like I was losing control of my own destiny.

Alex must have called Noreen that day, because she flew up from Florida the next. When she and Alex walked into the room, I was surprised to see her there. Noreen, always confident, always funny, and always brave, walked over to my bed with a big smile on her face, gave me a hug and a kiss, and demanded, as only a best friend can, "I didn't fly all this way to wait on you hand and foot. Now get your ass up out of that bed." All I could muster was, "Screw you." She laughed. I managed a chuckle.

I didn't know at the time that Alex had painted a ghastly picture of me during the drive from the airport to the hospital. When he warned Noreen that she wouldn't recognize me, she told him, "I'd recognize that girl with a bag over her head." In her mind, I could never look or be as sick as Alex described, and she felt a little angry with him for his portrayal of something that couldn't possibly be. Yet when she first saw me, asleep in bed, she later admitted that she saw the illness Alex had described, was seized by fear, and initially wanted to run away and pretend that none of this was happening. She then took a deep breath and began doing what she had flown all the way to do—and that was to be the best friend anyone could have.

I thank God for sending Noreen that week. Best friends hear everything you *don't* say. Sure, they're the ones who will leave a party with you when they're having fun and you're not. And they're the ones who will stay home with you until your bad haircut grows out. But no friend is ever prepared to support you, much less your spouse, through something as devastating as cancer.

Noreen flew twelve hundred miles to try, and she did one hell of a great job. She was my companion and my prop. She did countless things that said, "You aren't alone. You've got a big load, but I'm here to help you carry it." She screened phone calls, brought in whatever I wanted from home, fetched drinks. She let me whine a little, or a lot, and then made me walk—okay, shuffle—one more lap around the hall when I would rather have quit. She brought up only the old memories she knew would make me laugh, and she even helped me to laugh at myself.

Noreen never felt sorry for me, knowing that I could manufacture enough self-pity on my own. She never told me how brave or courageous I was, clearly understanding that I had never volunteered to have cancer. And never once did she say, "You'll be fine." Instead, she bemoaned my predicament with me. Most of all, she never feared saying the "wrong" thing. She simply was herself, and never was her friendship needed or appreciated more. Without her strength—and especially her humor—I might have lost all my weakened emotional equilibrium.

Alex, too, was glad Noreen had come. She became his assistant cheerleader who could stay with me when he couldn't. Still, he was torn between wanting to ignore everything except me and knowing that he had to keep the business afloat. Guilt gnawed at him when he wasn't by my side.

My second roommate arrived the same day Noreen did.

She was a spunky twenty-nine-year-old woman with lupus and bladder cancer and tubes and pain. She and I tried to keep our spirits up while our friends and family visited, but at night, in the darkness, we shared the common experience of cancer that only cancer patients can know. We talked about its indignities the way others might talk about the inconvenience of having a dead battery. She regretted that she would probably never marry and have children. Silently, I felt sorry for her and thanked my lucky stars that if cancer had to strike me, at least it had given me more years than she would probably ever see. When she casually and matter-of-factly brought up the subject of dying, I joined in the conversation without difficulty. For the first time in my life, I actually spoke, to an almost total stranger, about death—my own. It was deeply depressing.

Five days after entering what I had begun to call Hotel Hell, Dr. Kaminski reached into his arsenal and brought out a stronger chemotherapy called CHOP, which is CVP with the addition of Adriamycin, a drug which also interferes with DNA repair. I was to take it in eight three-week cycles, and I hoped it would work. If not, one of my options would be forever gone because CHOP is cardiotoxic and can only be administered once in a lifetime.

Wondering if CHOP would, in fact, be any more successful than CVP, I asked Dr. Kaminski, quite bluntly, to evaluate my odds. I should have known he was too smart to fall into that trap. With optimistic compassion, he simply answered, "We still have many options." I wanted him to be more specific, knowing fully that he couldn't. And regardless of what numbers he might have given me, my odds were still fifty-fifty. Sooner or later, lymphoma or a truck or plain old age would get me. How could I expect Dr. Kaminski to know what or when?

Alex stayed with me long after the first CHOP treatment was over. I was terribly groggy and remember little about his presence. Months later, he recalled sitting in the darkness of my room, his resolve to stay positive and strong shattered by the avalanche of complications I was suffering. He feared the worst, tried to believe the best, and finally decided it would be best not to feel. Anything. He told himself that he needed simply to exist in order to face potential subsequent setbacks. While he wanted to believe that each tomorrow would bring improvement, he could find no solid evidence on which to build that hope. CVP had failed. There was no guarantee that CHOP would succeed. What if it didn't?

Almost immediately, CHOP began to work nearly too well. Lickety-split, the cells that had been trying to kill me began to die, but they were dumping their contents into me faster than my kidneys could get rid of the waste. Even in death, those bad cells didn't want to surrender, I thought. Couldn't they just go away and leave me alone?

In order to counteract the renal failure that followed, Dr. Kaminski decided to blow me up like a balloon. Industrial strength Sani-Flush, otherwise known as saline, was aggressively pumped into me to flush out my kidneys, but my body could not eliminate the solution as quickly as it flowed into me. Within hours, my poor frame was stressed under the weight of about twenty extra pounds, pounds that stretched the skin on my thighs and abdomen so tight I thought it would rip. The bloat potion distributed excess weight evenly from my head to my feet—almost. The only place it missed was my chest, and Noreen and I had to laugh that not a single ounce found its way there. We considered scolding Dr. Kaminski for this oversight, but decided not to embarrass him.

At least that's what I'd thought until six months later when Noreen filled me in on what really happened. "There you were, half dead, and all you worried about was pumping up your boobs." Breaking into laughter, she added, "You gave Dr. Kaminski hell about it, too."

"No way," I insisted.

"Oh yeah, you kept telling him you wanted a vote in where you got pumped up."

"I *didn't* say that to him," I declared, twisting my face in disbelief.

"Oh, you *did*," she convinced me. I groaned, put my head in my hand, laughed with mild embarrassment, and persuaded myself that he has heard worse from other drug-drenched patients.

I may have been joking around that day, but Alex was at his wit's end. The news of renal failure annihilated whatever remaining control he had managed to maintain over his emotions. By the time he left the hospital that evening, he was distraught. At home, he and Noreen discussed the situation over a couple of drinks. Alex had far more than a couple, and I would eventually learn from both of them that alcohol and emotions and exhaustion fueled an argument that night.

Alex told Noreen he was glad she was there, but felt guilty about putting what he considered his responsibility on someone else. He couldn't understand why this was happening to him—or to me. It was so unfair. He felt burdened and isolated by an illness over which he had no control. And with complications striking one blow after another, how could he possibly manage the company, Zan, Greta, and life in general while finding the time and mental strength to support me? Finally, he lashed out at Noreen that she would be with me for a week, but that he would be stuck with the long-term consequences, whatever they may be. Wrestling with her own fears and thinking that Alex wouldn't be *stuck* with anything if I didn't pull out soon, she lashed back, "Alex, this isn't about you. It's about Betsy."

Angrily, Alex stormed out of the house. Noreen panicked, knowing that he shouldn't be driving, but unsure of where he might go and unfamiliar with Ann Arbor, she could do nothing but hope he would return safely—and soon. She went upstairs to bed, but lay awake in the darkness until she heard the back door bang shut. The following morning, they found Alex's truck parked at an angle partially on the driveway and partially on the grass. He had obviously stumbled out of the truck and left the door open, and the light had drained his battery. I shuddered when both Noreen and Alex later told me of this incident, and I thanked whatever angel had ridden with Alex that night.

Over coffee the next morning, both regretted their

argument. Noreen realized that Alex was struggling emotionally far more than I was. She couldn't solve all his fears, but she was somehow able to convince him to pull himself together. I think she acknowledged that he would indeed need to fall apart sometime, but that he and his strength needed to be there for me now.

Noreen also suggested ways for Alex to manage the day-to-day responsibilities. She pointed out that people truly wanted to help, but couldn't possibly know how unless he told them. She also tried to convince him that he didn't always need to be Zan's chauffer, and she assured him that it was okay to ask another parent to drive occasionally. She recommended that the next time someone offered to bring dinner, he could thank them and suggest the day that it would be most helpful. "What was the point in having five casseroles in one day?" she asked. And she teased, "Alex, you can run a company and ask a bank for hundreds of thousands of dollars. When someone offers to bring you dinner, surely you can tell him or her which day would be best." They laughed over these simple suggestions, none of which had ever occurred to him. Life's little simplicities would be difficult for my fiercely independent husband to implement, but he did learn, however slowly.

Noreen and Alex agreed to work together to help me heal, one small, specific step at a time. Dr. Kaminski wanted me up and walking, and Noreen would see to it that I did. He also wanted to make sure that I ate properly, so both would see to it that I had food that appealed to me. Little did they know that their resolution to champion my diet would be a monumental challenge. The medications had crippled my taste buds and perverted the normal flavor of all foods. Hospitals are not famous for fine cuisine, but the food became absolutely unbearable. Breakfast, lunch, and dinner smelled and looked repulsive. I was sure that the EPA had given the food a five-star rating—for toxic waste. I told Noreen they should give the recipes to pest control companies—it would kill anything.

Fortunately, there was a refrigerator in the lounge where patients could store food, so Noreen and Alex brought food from home, although it didn't taste much better than the hospital's. Nearly everything tasted like salt or metal, and I could scarcely bear to eat. By week's end, I could tolerate steak, steak, or steak and drink Coke, Coke, or Coke, though I had never been a big meat eater or soda drinker. It was simply all that would pass my throat without making me gag.

I had never considered myself particularly vain, but I learned in the hospital that indeed I was. My physical appearance reminded me that I was, in fact, ill. A friend's uncle, who was also a patient on the floor, mistook Noreen for my daughter. People used to mistake us for sisters. Bloated and pale, I did look horrible. Even if I had tried to wear makeup, nothing could have camouflaged my puffy face or widened the slits my eyes had become. I wanted no one to see me this way—not Alex, not Noreen, not a nurse, not a doctor. But what was a girl to do?

I was neither a pretty sight nor did I feel like being a pleasant hostess. Noreen and Alex did an outstanding job of discouraging people from visiting, thank goodness. I was too tired to talk to the people who called, much less to entertain visitors.

In my previous life, my daily routine had been anything but routine. Every day was a haphazard mix of meeting clients at jobsites, meeting potential clients at various properties, searching for specialty sinks or whatever else our clients could dream up, planning the next marketing blitz, and attending various meetings. Unfettered to any particular place, I moved about each and every day from half-built houses to clients' offices or homes to building suppliers, always remaining flexible enough to meet with a prospective client on short notice. In the hospital, I was separated from this ordinary life. Confined to half a room, dependent on drugs and oxygen, I was robbed of my health, my freedom, and, I feared, my future.

The world outside my hospital room was going on without me. As chair of the Sales and Marketing Council of the local Home Builders Association, I should have been at the biggest event of the year, but it took place without me. And when Alex sold one of our homes late in the week, I should have been happy, but I felt cheated out of doing my job. *I* sold our homes. *He* built them. That's the way things were supposed to be. But my condition had put an end to that, and I hated my body for its utter failure.

And did I mention the hospital's idea of a hat? It's a plastic contraption that looks like an upside down Stetson, neatly fits over the throne, and catches human waste. After my kidneys failed, I got my own hat, after which my rectal and urethral activities became news to all, much to my embarrassment. Every fluid ounce that came out of me got trapped in that hat, measured, and recorded. I think all the patients on the floor had their own hats. At least my nose suggested that frequent flushing was not an option.

When I filled the hat to the proper line, the aides and nurses cheered as if I were two years old and had just gone "pee-pee" in the potty for the first time. I knew they were just trying to encourage me, but their reactions were puzzling. I simply could not imagine measuring and recording human waste, let alone getting excited about it. What a nasty job. Juli assured me that no one in a hospital thinks anything of it, but I did.

The IVs were regularly changed in order to avoid infection at any given site, and my blood was drawn twice daily. There were so many holes in me that I was sure I would spring a leak. And just what did the hospital do with all the blood it amassed? Noreen and I were sure that secret pagan rituals were being held somewhere.

Early each morning, Grand Marshal Dr. Kaminski led a parade of four or five residents into my room. Together, they listened to my heart and lungs, looked at whatever part of me they wanted to see, assessed the previous day and night's developments, and planned whatever remedies they deemed appropriate for the upcoming day and night. During the parade, the residents always walked quietly in perfect step behind the grand marshal. But when he was back in the clinic or the classroom or wherever his schedule took him, one or another of the residents returned later in the day and evening. And it was then that they weren't so quiet. In fact, they let their personalities shine brightly.

Young, brilliant, enthusiastic, and excited about their budding careers, the residents reminded me of puppies on puppy chow. One glowed when he spoke of his soon-to-be bride, and I couldn't help but smile with him. Early one morning, another slipped quietly into my room, saw tears falling from my closed eyes, sat in the chair beside my bed, and lifted my hand gently before I even knew she was there.

It occurred to me that these residents had nearly completed grueling training in the latest and greatest medical techniques and therapies, but they were still reporting to a grand marshal, otherwise known as an attending physician. Teaching hospitals are much too modest about this service, and I thought about offering to write a free ad campaign for them. The headline would read, "Huge Sale on Medical Services. Buy 4—Sometimes 5 or 6—Geniuses for The Price of 1!" In a teaching hospital, that's exactly what you get—doctors who check on you not just once a day, but several times. It's the best deal around.

And the nurses? They not only faithfully carried out the doctors' orders, but also took the time to make small talk, a gesture that seemingly recognized me as a human being with a life outside the hospital. Every one of them gave me an extra dose of kindness along with the medications they administered.

Claudia, coordinator of the support group, stopped by periodically with magazines and uplifting words. Judy, too, brought her caring gentleness which I had come to know so well. Both always sensed my frame of mind immediately and knew exactly what to say to make certain that they left me feeling more upbeat than they found me.

By week's end, I desperately wanted Alex to hold me close, and when he still didn't, I assumed that he was repulsed by my appearance and felt awkward coming near me and my tubes. Even in my drugged stupor, I could clearly see that he was physically exhausted and emotionally drained, and I felt terrible for causing him so much stress. Lightly, I reminded him to get a full medical report on anyone he dated after I was gone. He simply shook his head and stared blankly back at me.

Many months later, I asked Alex how much my physical appearance had repulsed him. "It didn't in the slightest," he replied.

"Right," I sarcastically shot back.

"Repulse is the wrong word," he reflected. "Your physical appearance told me how sick you were. I was never repulsed by it. I was scared to death, and if I'd crawled onto your bed and held you in my arms, I'd have lost it—and *that* was the last thing you needed."

That was a big admission from someone who rarely expresses his feelings, and I replied, "If I'm ever in that condition again, will you skip the macho stuff and just hold me?" He promised he would.

By the end of the first week, I began to lobby aggressively to go home. Like a spoiled child, I repeatedly begged Dr. Kaminski to release me, and like a patient parent, he repeatedly explained that my blood counts and creatinine levels had to normalize first. If I had been in his shoes, I might have screamed at me, "What part of 'no' don't you understand?"

As I entered that second weekend in Hotel Hell, I was desperate for fresh air. On Saturday, I begged Alex to smuggle me out, just for an hour, to take me for a ride anywhere. He wouldn't have, of course, but his excuse was that we couldn't fit the IV pole in the car. I moaned that I would hold it out the window. When Dr. Kaminski visited, I jokingly threatened to break a window if I couldn't breathe some air soon. The good doctor gave me a pass to walk to the courtyard. Walk? Given the size of the hospital complex, the courtyard was much too far to walk to in my condition. Noreen immediately rounded up a wheelchair, returned to my room with it, offered me a chariot ride, and with IV pole in tow, pushed me to freedom, or at least as much freedom as I had known in a week. Outside, I took a deep breath, and the fragrance of spring flowers and fresh grass was intoxicating, not to mention a welcome change from the waste-tainted air I'd been breathing for seven days.

Noreen spread a sheet on the grass and we sprawled out to sunbathe just as we had so often done in years past. Only in years past, we had sunbathed in bikinis, poolside or at the ocean's edge. Now, I sported pajamas and a terry bathrobe, and the tube between my arm and the IV pole barely stretched long enough to allow me to lie down. I jested to Noreen, "Weird tan lines, huh?"

We may not have been exactly the bathing beauties we had once fancied ourselves, but the sun warmed my body and spirit. As I looked around at other patients in their own wheelchairs and bathrobes, attached to their own IV poles, I couldn't help but observe, "This scene is straight out of *One Flew Over the Cuckoo's Nest*. What the hell are *we* doing here?" How far we had come from our younger, carefree days.

By Sunday, my crisis was subsiding, and Alex stayed home to work on one of his old Jaguars, an overdue diversion he rarely permits himself even in the best of times, but one which he now desperately needed. I missed him terribly. Noreen and I spent the day sunbathing, watching movies, and monitoring my counts. Late in the afternoon, Alex, Ted, and Lisa brought dinner, and we all picnicked in the courtyard.

Close to midnight that night, I was hungry. My pole and I lumbered to the lounge to retrieve some of my morsels from the refrigerator. Even if food tasted terrible, I presumed that hunger was a good sign. On the way, I passed a door on which a large, handwritten note hung. It said, "No crying allowed." The patient inside was dying, and I had no way of knowing that his daughter and son-in-law were sleeping in the lounge. Only they weren't exactly sleeping. When I flipped on the light, I found them on the couch making love. I don't know who was more embarrassed, but I returned to my room as quickly as I could plod down the hall. Hungry and envious, I crawled into my own bed, tearfully aching for Alex. The Invisible Invader had long since clobbered our own intimacy.

In the darkness, a thousand what-ifs cluttered my

thoughts. I was no longer the person Alex had fallen in love with, much less married. Would he have fallen in love with me knowing I had lymphoma? Of course not, I decided. What appeal did I have left? None. I had become everything I had never wanted to be.

And what if I didn't recover? I didn't want Alex to spend the rest of his life alone. I wanted him to spend it with *me*, not with some other woman. The tears I shed that night could have created a whole new body of water. It might have been called "The Sea of Self-Pity."

At last, on Memorial Day morning, Dr. Kaminski released me from Hotel Hell. That name was a reflection of my own frustrations, not of the people who worked there. If I had named it for them, it would have been Paradise Palace or something equally complimentary. Without a doubt, every person—from the doctors to the residents to the nurses to the aides—did his or her best to treat me in the most humane and respectful way. None of them ever treated me as an object or as a task to be completed. Instead, all seemed acutely aware that their tenderness made a palpable difference in my comfort, if not my recovery. I saw a glowing halo over the head of each person who assisted in my care. Their extraordinary kindness helped me to maintain some measure of sanity.

When I reflect back on my hospital stay, I realize that I was at least drugged much of the time. Alex and Noreen had faced reality cold. It takes an enormous amount of stamina and courage for anyone to sit in a hospital room day after day, watching a loved one in such a frail condition.

Alex did the best he could, but each of my physical failures had tightened the emotional noose around his neck. Noreen, thankfully, did the best she could to loosen it, but it would take some time for him to breathe comfortably again.

Despite Alex, Noreen, and the remarkable hospital staff, I had simply become a caged animal. I'd endured ten days of boredom, punctuated by fear and self-pity. I'd wondered if I would ever reclaim my ordinary life. Did I dare to expect the CHOP to succeed? And a future? I wasn't even certain I'd be around to wear the summer sandals I had bought on sale the previous winter. My confidence in everything had fallen to zero. I knew I was lucky to leave the hospital in one piece. I'd had no surgery or any other far worse procedure. My body was intact, but the rest of me felt like it had been mortally wounded.

CHAPTER EIGHT

FROM MISERABLE TO MANGY

Returning home was like going to the Ritz. Never mind that housekeeping had overlooked the place for a couple of weeks. Not that Alex hadn't tried to straighten up, but how many hours are there in the day after working, preparing my takeout meals, and visiting the sick ward? To me, home looked like a palace, Tooties and I were overjoyed at our reunion, and I could get back to life.

Memorial Day, my first day home, was gloriously bright and sunny. While Alex worked on his old car, Noreen drove us around town to see the spring flowers which had blossomed during my incarceration. I'm sure she was happy to see some of the sights in Ann Arbor other than the hospital. Late in the afternoon, Lisa, Ted, and other friends stopped by for a cookout and to celebrate my release. Still bloated, my wardrobe was limited to stretch pants, but that mattered little.

I hadn't had a decent night's sleep in ten days, and by the end of the day, I was deliriously overjoyed to crawl high up into our antique double bed. I had hoped that Alex would hold me close in the darkness. Instead, he immediately fell asleep on his own side of the bed. Continents, rather than inches, seemed to separate us.

Alex *was* truly worn out. Months later, he would tell me that he had been the leader of my emotional battle as well as everyone else's—self-appointed, of course. When his parents and children, my sister and daughter and other friends had worried about me during my hospitalization, he had considered it his job to keep everyone focused on a positive outcome. He had repeatedly assured them that losing a battle didn't mean we were losing the war. Even though the war wasn't going according to plan, he had tried to convince them that my complications were only a temporary setback.

Alex hadn't, however, fully believed his own words, and he'd withdrawn further into himself searching for hope and strength and a remedy for his own wounds. Of course he was relieved that my hospital stay was over, but it had traumatized him so deeply that his raw emotions would require time to heal, just as my body did. At least he broke off his relationship with Jack Daniels.

Noreen returned to Florida the day after my release, and I returned to the couch—again. I slept and slept, and when I was awake, all I wanted to do was sleep.

At the end of the week, Alex and I would celebrate our birthdays. We were born three years and one day apart, but we'd grown up celebrating birthdays very differently. To me, birthdays are important rituals which celebrate each year of life. To Alex, birthdays are reminders of aging. I always had difficulty understating his birthday to his satisfaction, and he never managed to do enough on mine. Both of us usually got it wrong and managed to offend each other.

Alex's birthday arrived three days after my release, and we returned to Dr. Kaminski and Judy that day. I was utterly exhausted, and frustrated that my body had not let me return to normal living the minute I'd left the hospital. Judy voiced concern that I might be depressed. Who? Me? Of course not. Despite my vow to recognize and seek help for depression should it occur, I couldn't see the forest for the trees.

Physically, I was anemic. CHOP had wiped out not only the cancer cells but also the healthy cells that our bodies need to function properly. I was transferred to the infusion area where, for the next several hours, some healthy stranger's blood would, hopefully, jumpstart my body from its inertia. We arrived home well past dinner. A single candle pushed into a cookie made a poor substitute for the cake I had wanted to bake for Alex that day, but at least Zan and I sang "Happy Birthday" and gave him our presents and cards. For the first time, Alex's birthday was low-key, but another day at the hospital gave him no reason to believe that recovery was imminent. He wondered if it was even possible.

The following day—Friday, May 31—I turned fifty-two years old and spent most of the day dozing on the couch and looking forward to Alex coming home. More than any year before, I was thankful to be alive and thrilled to *have* a birthday. Alex got it all wrong. At least I thought he did.

Unquestionably, I was in no shape to do anything, but I had thought of suggesting that we all go out for ice cream after dinner. However, I never got the chance to bring it up. I was on the phone with Juli when Alex motioned that he was going shopping with Zan and a friend who was spending the night. They quickly disappeared before I could collect my thoughts. It was my birthday, for pete's sake, and he was taking the boys where? And leaving me behind to rot on the couch? I hated that couch, and no matter how hard it might be to unglue me from it, I wanted to get out of the house.

It was around ten o'clock by the time they returned home. He and the boys reported their outing which had included stopping for ice cream. And then Alex went to bed, but not before handing me a note which said, "I give you my karma. Happy Birthday." I was furious. No, I was seething. I had wanted to celebrate life, and they had left me out completely. And all I got was a handwritten note giving me that which cannot be given away? Never mind that Alex does have good karma. He's the luckiest man alive. If he were a rooster in a hen house, I am sure he would lay eggs. But was there something wrong with a tangible gift, even if it cost fifty cents? Did Alex think that spending even a penny was senseless if I were just going to die?

Well, I wasn't going to die, and I *was* going to enjoy at least some familiar birthday ritual, even if I had to do it all by myself. But how? For the first time in two weeks, I got in my car and drove around the neighborhood for a little while. When I got home, I placed a candle into another cookie, and then, in a pathetic act of self-pity, took it into our bedroom where Alex was sleeping and woke him up by singing "Happy Birthday to Me." Sleepily, he said nothing more than "What are you doing?" before rolling over and going back to sleep. Oh, how very sensitive. I might have entitled that night in our life, "Crazed Former Inmate Goes Berserk."

I sobbed myself to sleep on the couch that night and was not exactly happy the next morning. Alex couldn't understand why. He insisted that he had asked me if I wanted to go out for ice cream and that I had declined. Since I had seemed so tired, he thought it would be good to get the boys out of the house so that I could rest. Anyway, his mother was planning a birthday dinner for us both on Sunday. What was a couple of days?

In retrospect, and knowing Alex, he probably did mention ice cream, and given my dopey state of mind, I probably didn't remember—which of course makes me look like the self-absorbed prima donna that I was. Whichever it was, I pouted for a couple of days before finally realizing that Alex has never done a malicious thing in his life. And we did have a birthday party two days later, through which I mostly slept.

One week later, Alex's dad Ted turned ninety. Months earlier, we had planned a surprise party for him at our house. Some of his out-of-state friends were planning to make the trip. We had also invited several of our friends, younger of course than Ted, but whose company he thoroughly enjoyed. In my condition, however, I had no idea how I was going to host that party. Alex had called our friends while I was in the hospital and asked each of them to prepare a dish. All I had to do was straighten and decorate the house.

During the next week, I did a little housekeeping—a little—each day. In my previous life, I had been able to blitz through the house from top to bottom in no time. I suppose I could have hired help, but that would have meant admitting my own frailty. Forcing myself to get up and perform even mundane chores boosted my spirits and probably my energy. And Alex and Zan pitched in, as they always do.

My body also deflated slightly each day so that by week's end, I could squeeze into most of my wardrobe. I resembled my old self—sort of.

The afternoon of June 8 arrived, and guests filled our home for the first time in months. The table was laden with delicious food, and the house was at least presentable. When Ted arrived, he was taken aback by the presence of so many familiar faces, gathered to honor his long and healthy life. It was a lovely party, one which he thoroughly enjoyed.

Two days later, I was scheduled to receive my first treatment of Rituxan, a monoclonal antibody which is a man-made copy of antibodies normally secreted by white blood cells, specifically, lymphocytes. Rituxan binds to the surface antigen CD20 on the cancerous cells and causes them to burst. Adding Rituxan to chemotherapy has proven very promising.

Benadryl, administered prior to Rituxan in order to counteract potential flu-like symptoms, made me quite sleepy. About halfway through the infusion, I did develop a fever and chills, expected side effects often associated with the first Rituxan treatment. Judy immediately came to check on me, interrupted the infusion, ordered other drugs to offset the symptoms, and then restarted the Rituxan when they subsided. Hours later, I went home. Two days later, the second CHOP treatment would hopefully slaughter more cancer cells.

Still trying desperately to regain energy and strength two and half weeks after my release, I'd earned the title "Champion Couch Potato of the World." I simply could not make it through a day without napping, sometimes in the mornings, sometimes in the afternoons, often both. How could I plan a meeting or anything else without having confidence in my ability to perform the simple task of staying awake?

And then there was Alex, always ready, willing, and able to take me to whatever appointment or test I had. Always willing to cook dinner, do the laundry, and make the phone calls I should have made. And lately, always remote. It wasn't that he was ever mean-spirited. He simply moved about in a trance, his eyes hollow and his smile but a memory. I was somewhat aware of his own anxiety at the time, but too overwhelmed by my own to offer support. Sometimes I felt like we were on different planets.

Alex needed a break from this nightmare as much as I did, and fortunately one was approaching. For fourteen years, during the third week in June, he had taken the kids to Camp Michigania, a camp in northern Michigan for U of M alumni and their families. I was unable to go, but there was no reason for him or the kids to miss out. He looked forward to sailing, and the week at camp had always recharged his batteries. Would it have the same effect this year or was this year's stress simply too much to overcome in one week?

Alex had called Karen while I was in the hospital and had asked if she would stay with me during the week he would be at camp. When he had asked, Mother was also in the hospital, although she did not tell him—or me. At the time, she had feared losing us both but had promised him she would come. With the weight of a different world on her shoulders, she must have certainly wondered how she would manage to be there for me and our mother at the same time.

By the time Karen was to babysit me, Mother felt well enough to come along. She's always recovered remarkably quickly when her heart goes haywire, and her ninety-two-year-old heart had recovered faster than my fifty-two-year-old body. She and Karen arrived two days before Alex left for camp. By that time, I was certain I could have stayed alone, but knowing that I was in good hands if I needed them, Alex could leave guilt-free, and I was happy for the company.

Before he left, we hugged, holding each other closer than we had in weeks. Still, it was clear to me that while our bodies were close, we were separated by our own private agonies. This trip, I hoped, would restore his energy and improve his outlook. While he was gone, I vowed to try even harder to regain my own energy and to reclaim my optimism.

Earlier in the year, with the help of a good dictionary, I had fumbled my way through Medicalese, a prerequisite for understanding any medical malfunction, and I had managed to translate most of the medical jargon into plain English. "Bilateral axillary lymphadenopathy," for example, meant that the lymph nodes in both armpits were swollen. I guessed that my "shoddy inguinal" nodes meant that the nodes in my groin were of inferior quality. I wondered whose bad idea it was to make the language of medicine so complicated. Didn't the people responsible for naming medical malfunctions realize that having a disease is hard enough without having to wade through a terminology quagmire, or that puzzling terminology can make patients feel more like victims of disease rather than beneficiaries of miraculous medicine? Maybe I could teach them a lesson by rewriting Builderese specifically for health care professionals. Imagine the puzzled looks I would get when I asked for their choice of "conflagrated terra" when all I really meant was bricks? I chuckled at the thought of such sweet revenge.

One word, "alopecia," particularly amused me. In Medicalese, it means baldness. What a melodious word for such a malevolent malady. For kicks, when my hair began to fall out the very day Alex left, I looked up the word in the dictionary, only to find that its Greek root, "alopekia," means "fox mange." I swear I didn't make that up. Well, I was about to become mangy, and you can just imagine how much that self-perception bolstered my spirits.

About four hours after Alex left, alopecia struck without warning. In the kitchen, I was slicing peaches into a bowl when I thought I caught a glimpse of something falling past my right eye. Something was falling, all right—*my hair.* A few strands hit the counter, but most landed in the bowl atop the peaches. Without thinking, I laid down the knife and grabbed my head, whereupon my scalp surrendered more hair to my sticky, juice-covered hand. Kinda gives new meaning to peach fuzz, doesn't it?

I wanted to scream. But Mother and Karen were nearby, and I really didn't want to share that moment with anyone. So I screamed silently—very loudly. Fortunately, they were watching a movie with their backs turned to me. Quietly, I pitched the hairy concoction, wrapped a kitchen towel around my head so that I wouldn't leave a trail, and escaped upstairs unnoticed.

In the bathroom, I couldn't help but stare at the bald spot. It looked weird, and I grimaced. I also made several primeval groans before deciding that temporary baldness was a small price to pay for my life. I then slipped a knit cap over my head to catch the mess and returned downstairs as if nothing had happened.

For five days thereafter, my hair vigorously deserted my scalp. In the garage each morning, I leaned over the garbage can and brushed out clumps of hair. Then, after showering, I removed more locks from the drain. By day and by night, the knit cap contained the evidence of uncontrollable shedding. On the sixth morning, when I brushed what little remained attached to my scalp, the last vestiges stubbornly stayed in place. They were taunting reminders of what had once covered my head. So much for having bad hair days. They'd all be bad for quite some time.

I'd planned to shave what little hair remained that day but decided I would wait to see just how much more deserted me. None did. The Great Hair Loss was over. In the mirror, I looked at the few wisps that remained and thought, "Yeah, this *does* look like I have mange. Good thing Dr. Kaminski became a physician. He'd have made a lousy hairdresser," an observation I jokingly shared with him some weeks later. Whoever chose that alopecia word hit the nail on the head, pun intended.

Karen was fascinated by my loss. It exposed the big red birthmarks on the back of my scalp, and she remarked with a laugh, "Wow, I haven't seen those in fifty-two years." I replied, "I could have done without seeing them at all." She wanted to take a picture, but I refused. Mange was outward evidence of my interior malfunction, and I did not need a permanent impression for something that I was trying to believe was only temporary. More than ever before, I needed reminders of the normal me, and I was turning anywhere I could to find them, including dabbing shampoo on my nearly naked noggin. A girl can pretend, can't she?

Mother knew I was losing my hair but still did not associate it with chemotherapy or cancer. She once asked if my blood disorder had a name and I answered that it was called follicular lymphoma. Just as I knew she would, she replied, "Oh, I'll never remember that."

Mother, Karen, and I had never spent time alone together without husbands and children, and we had an enjoyable visit despite the fact that we did absolutely nothing of any consequence. Our only outings were to the hospital for blood tests and to the grocery store. Mother was quite content to read or watch TV, although, even with hearing aids, the decibel level at which she listened to the TV almost propelled Karen and me to another planet. I, too, was content to do no more than was absolutely necessary. Each afternoon, Mother and I invariably dozed. Karen must have been bored out of her wits, but she hid it well.

One evening when Juli called, she spoke with Karen, and obviously asked how I was *really* doing. Karen wandered into another room where she thought I wouldn't hear and told Juli, "Your mother looks like she just got out of Auschwitz." I pretended not to hear, but I wanted to walk into the other room and ask Karen, "When did you say your plane was leaving?" Did I really look that awful? I guess I had thinned down. I'd lost more pounds than Dr. Kaminski's bloat potion had ever put on me, and it would take some time for me to eat enough to regain my normal weight.

As the older sister, Karen could easily have babied me that week. Thankfully, she didn't. Like Noreen had been, she was simply herself and treated me as if nothing were different. While she'd offer to help with dinner, she never insisted on cooking for us. She must have instinctively known that letting me perform even simple tasks would help me regain my independence and confidence. Big Sister even let me put the dishes in the dishwasher.

Fortunately, Karen watched out for me without smothering me. When I decided to bake a ham at the end of the week, just before Alex was to return, Karen quietly removed it from the oven just after I placed it in. She'd noticed that

I had left the wrapper on it, even while scoring and inserting cloves into it. "Oh gosh," she said lightly. "We were gabbing away and I just noticed this." I felt like a complete idiot, but she laughed it off and sweetly assured me, "We were just paying too much attention to our conversation. Anybody could have done it." No, just someone with the beginning of chemo brain, a side effect that reduces concentration and mental clarity.

Preparing meals for the three of us did not exactly require much effort. Mother preferred simple meals and very little on her plate. Karen was content with anything. And my taste buds were beginning to recover, but were nowhere near normal. When Mother and Karen first arrived, I was still consuming an all-meat diet. Throughout their visit, I added a little rice, a little salad—and peaches. Oh, how I devoured sweet, juicy peaches. Except, of course, the two that had served as the landing deck for my hair.

One evening, while I was standing at the kitchen sink peeling peaches, Mother slowly sauntered over, put her hand on my shoulder and offered these words of wisdom: "You know, peaches are a lot like life. Peel off the unimportant things, throw away the pits, and you have sweet fruit." Hmm. She's right, I thought. Oh, how I desperately wanted to pitch the pits and taste life's sweetness again.

Alex called several times a day, and each day he sounded more and more relaxed. I missed him terribly, but was happy that he was taking a well-deserved break from work—and from the Invisible Invader. Toward the end of the week, he laughed when I warned him to prepare himself for a mangy wife, and when I told him alopecia's root meant fox mange, he replied that I was dwelling on the wrong part. "Forget about the mange. I think you're a fox." I was totally taken aback by this mildly flirtatious response, the first I could remember since my diagnosis. I don't remember what I said, but I do remember thinking that he just hadn't seen me yet, and that I wished I could live up to that expectation.

I spent a little extra time getting ready the morning Alex was due home. I just wanted to look like—*be* like—my old self. The wig—I remembered the wig. First I put on the stocking, a wig undergarment which made me look like I was about to rob a bank, and then pulled on the wig, which looked like bad faux fur to me. It wasn't a thing like my hair, but it might help me feign resemblance to the old me.

Dressed at last, I went downstairs where Mother and Karen were already getting their breakfast. "Oh, you look so cute," they said. "The wig is great, and you can't even tell it's a wig." Maybe they couldn't tell, but I could. Even if it had looked exactly like my hair, it felt completely different. Its elastic band gripped my scalp like a vice, and I was quite certain that at any moment this faux fur was going to pop straight from the top of my head like a champagne cork.

I was as ready as I could be for Alex's homecoming later that morning. Tanned and smiling, he pulled into the driveway a week after he had left. Thankfully, his hug left no doubt that he had missed me and that his spirit was renewed. Still, I wondered how he would react to my head, so I stripped the wig shortly after his arrival. Without blinking an eye, he pulled me close to him and said, "You look beautiful." I love it when he lies.

Months later, when I asked him how he had *really* felt about my head, he assured me that he had never cared whether I had hair or not. Hair loss was simply part of the treatment, it was temporary, and it seemed so insignificant compared to what I had gone through in the hospital. "I was just glad you were alive and getting better. I knew your hair would grow back. Your life wouldn't," he said.

Mother and Karen returned to Virginia two days after Alex came home. Never before had I cherished their companionship so deeply. Although my mother's diminished comprehension prevented me from drawing on her emotional strength, I knew that her ninety-two-year-old genes resided in me, and against odds of her own, her continued presence in this world gave me great hope. And *that* was more encouraging than any words she could have said in her younger years.

I'd expected to return directly home after taking Mother and Karen to the airport, but Judy called just as I was getting in my car. My neutrophils were down again, and she wanted me to start taking Neupogen. Would it be possible, she asked, for me to come to the clinic? "I'm on my way," I said, wondering all the way there how I would cross this next hurdle.

CHAPTER NINE

THE SUMMER OF OBLIVION

Neupogen is a drug which raises the neutrophil count, and I'd have taken anything to avoid risking another stay in Hotel Hell, but there was a big problem. Neupogen was given by injection—self-injection. How was a yellow-bellied, chicken-hearted milksop like me supposed to jab herself with a razor-sharp instrument? I got lightheaded just thinking about it. Maybe it would come with a chaser of smelling salts.

Dr. Kaminski's nurse, Sandy Trembath, would teach me how to administer the shots. When I told her that I had failed masochist school, she promised to give them to me herself if I couldn't. I loved her for giving me that safety net, but I agreed to try. She then asked me to watch a video about Neupogen and self-injections, which I did—three times. Following along with the tape, I pinched my thigh in preparation for the poke and used my fingernail to pretend I was puncturing the skin. But just before the actual penetration, my tummy turned somersaults, and my eyes involuntarily turned away.

At the end of the tape, the spokesperson said, "Congratulations for participating in your care." She sounded so smug that I retorted in frustration, "I'm *not* going to participate in this particular part of my care. What are *you* gonna do about it, lady?" Before returning to Sandy, I called Alex, asked if he would lend his bravery to a worthy cause, and he reluctantly promised to try. Sandy gave me the shot that day. Alex and I would return the following afternoon for his lesson.

I knew that Alex was a little squeamish about shots, but since he'd once planned to become a surgeon, I assumed that he knew he would have had to inflict gruesome gashes, far more invasive than these needles—which were, in truth, almost miniscule. But when Sandy tried to hand him the syringe, he involuntarily stepped back from it and every bit of color faded from his face. Sandy patiently suggested that he watch while she gave me the shot. Like me, he turned his head at the moment of penetration. It was clear that he was no better at this than I. Sandy never made us feel like the sissies we were, but I knew Alex's pride was wounded. I promised Sandy I could find people to give me the shots and we left.

On the way home, Alex's face reflected disappointment in his failure to perform what seemed like such a simple task. He finally admitted, "I'm afraid I'll hurt you." Touched by his tenderness, I tried hard to assure him that giving shots was hard for many people, that it wasn't necessary for him to do everything for me, and that he shouldn't be embarrassed or ashamed of it. Our friend Marie the dentist gave me the injections for the remainder of the week, and she never made fun of Alex or me.

For the next couple of months, blood was extracted every Monday and every Thursday. Although I tired of stretching out my arm for modern day vampires to suck out my blood, those nurses were the sweetest vampires I have ever met. They were well aware that their cancer patients were in serious medical trouble, but their smiles, their friendly manners, and their encouraging words maintained a positive, upbeat atmosphere in the blood drawing area. Most importantly, those internal audits kept Dr. Kaminski, Judy, and me well-acquainted with whatever fickle notions my blood might be entertaining. And how badly could it damage me between those frequent audits?

Despite taking Neupogen and the regular blood draws, I was preoccupied with infection and afraid that my body was defenseless against relentlessly attacking germs which might send me straight back to Hotel Hell. Since my release, I had washed my hands constantly, fearing that germs were crawling all over them. When I couldn't wash them, I used antibacterial wipes. Tasting germs in every bite, I washed food until it was barely recognizable, even before cooking it. We stopped going out to restaurants for fear that germs lurked in their kitchens. On the handles of grocery carts, on my steering wheel, on doorknobs, I imagined a microscopic army plotting to invade my body. Germs were everywhere, and they made life itself a danger. I became a virtual exile, preferring to stay at home unless it was absolutely necessary to go out.

Fortunately, I could work mostly at home and by phone.

By early July, when the third CHOP treatment and the second Rituxan treatment were administered on the same day, I was tired, but could stay awake throughout almost every day. Chemo brain, however, had already begun, and it would throw me into cognitive bondage for the next few months, although I wasn't even aware that I'd been captured. I knew only that I was having difficulty remembering even some of the simplest things.

Still, I really did want to work, and Alex encouraged me to do as much as I felt I could. I'd schedule meetings with clients or prospective clients, and I found it uncanny that, on one pretense or another, he just happened to drop by during my meetings. It would take me months to figure out that he was giving me just enough room to regain my confidence without giving me any room to fall flat on my face. Pretty good guy, huh?

In truth, I was barely competent. Our building contracts, which at one time I knew backward and forward, became unfamiliar. When prospective clients asked about change orders, I fumbled through the pages looking for the appropriate paragraph, instead of reciting the contract language while referring them to paragraph fourteen, page three. And I could barely calculate the math, regardless of how simple it was. A 500,000 dollar purchase with a 100,000 dollar deposit left what balance? I would stare at the figures and eventually use a calculator to determine it.

My attempts at client selections were worse. Our purchasing agent ordered all materials directly from selection forms, and I had always been extremely careful to submit them accurately. One transposed number could mean very unhappy clients if pink carpet were installed instead of beige. When I submitted a selection form with two different tiles for the same fireplace, we all realized that my remaining brain cells should be added to the endangered species list. Alex began to double-check all my work.

And I should have been proactively marketing our properties more aggressively than ever, but I rarely gave it a thought. And oblivious to time, deadlines for selections came and went, and I simply forgot that the office needed to purchase materials by specific dates in order to maintain the flow of construction. Although Alex had no spare time to tackle one more task, he somehow picked up that slack, too, although I was relatively unaware of it at the time.

Fortunately for me, Mystic Ridge, the large project we had hoped to begin in the spring, had been delayed. By summer, when final details were being worked out, I was already behind in developing the marketing materials. I tried, but I would simply stare at the computer screen for hours and draw a complete blank. Not good for someone who had once been able to write marketing materials effortlessly. Eventually, I got it done, but it's a good thing Alex didn't pay me by the hour.

I am very lucky that neither our purchasing agent nor Alex were ever critical, at least not to my face. Of course, they were both in awkward positions. How could Alex replace his wife in the middle of her battle with cancer? And how could an employee criticize the boss's wife? I'm sure their patience stretched awfully thin sometimes.

Much later, Alex admitted that my diminished mental faculties did frustrate him at times, and that occasionally he had to remind himself that chemo brain was only a temporary side effect. "But mostly," he said, "I saw your efforts and interest as an encouraging sign of your determination to maintain a normal life. And if you made a few mistakes or were a little too slow along the way, I much preferred your making attempts to making none at all."

Alex also told me that I had asked him for help on a number of occasions and that he had thought that I must be improving if I could recognize my own fogginess. Funny, I don't remember asking him for a single thing.

In early July, our friend Dan died of liver cancer. He'd only been diagnosed a month and a half earlier. Dan was Alex's lumber salesman, and we knew him professionally more than personally. Still, he and I had spoken about our cancers, and his quick death frightened me. His funeral scared the hell out of me.

After the service, Alex and I made a quick stop at the hardware store. Standing behind us at the cash register, a distinguished looking gentlemen, in his mid-seventies perhaps, said to me, "Excuse me, but I couldn't help but notice your hat. It's lovely, and you don't often see such elegance these days."

I have no idea how I responded to that stranger. I hope I thanked him, but chemo may very well have destroyed my etiquette cells. It didn't destroy my anger. When Alex and I got into the car moments later, I burst into tears and sobbed, "I hate this hat. If my body hadn't betrayed me, I wouldn't be wearing it."

Startled by my reaction, Alex tried to help me look at the brighter side. "Betsy, the compliment should make you happy. You look great today, and you're hiding the illness well."

"I don't want to hide anything," I cried, "and I don't want to be sick." I was inconsolable.

That night, when I asked Alex if he would promise to cremate me, he furrowed his eyebrows and sighed, "Betsy, you're going to be around for a long time. You shouldn't worry yourself about that."

"I'm not worried. Just promise you'll burn me," I said.

His face contorted as he replied, "Betsy, I don't even want to talk about this. And why do you have to be so blunt?"

"Well, talking about it isn't going to kill either of us. And burning's what it is. So please just promise."

Alex finally shut me up by saying, "I think you'll outlive me. But if you promise to cremate me, I'll cremate you if anything happens to you first." We had a deal. It was the first time we had mentioned death, at least that I remembered, and I knew when to stop. I didn't dare ask him to scatter my ashes in the ocean.

From that day forward and for the next several weeks, my car and I made an unusual detour whenever I drove to our downtown office, which I occasionally visited for various reasons. The most direct route took me directly past Muehlig Funeral Chapel where Dan's funeral had been held, but I could no longer drive past the place without envisioning my remains in some little urn. I began to take a different route, as if I could avoid the urn by avoiding the building.

By mid-July, just prior to the fourth CHOP and third Rituxan treatment, Alex and I were thrilled that another CT scan indicated good resolution of the disease. At last the toxins were winning. I began to allow myself to think—a little—about life after chemo. Maybe, just maybe, life would someday return to normal.

Alex and I celebrated by taking a Saturday day trip. We packed a cooler and drove north, stopping at a public beach and wading along the shore of Lake Huron. I had longed to be in Florida with Juli and the babies, but didn't dare set foot in a germ-infested airplane. I had longed, too, for the ocean, but had satisfied that desire by holding a conch shell to my ear and pretending that the waves were lapping at my feet. Lake Huron was as close as I was going to get to any large body of water that summer, and I giggled with delight when I wiggled my toes in the water.

We nearly left cancer in Ann Arbor for the entire day, referring to it only once when I told Alex that I wanted to leave something permanent for the people I love. Should I paint something special for him? Write a poem? What would he like? His face told me that he wished I hadn't brought up any reference to my possible demise, but without hesitation he said, "You already gave me something permanent. My wedding ring."

This wasn't a typical wedding ring. It was a signet ring emblazoned with his family's coat-of-arms. For years, I'd heard about a similar ring which had belonged to his father, and which had been stolen some twenty-five years earlier during a robbery in Alex's house shortly after Ted had given it to him. I'd never known Alex to wear jewelry, not even a watch, but that ring was obviously sentimental to him. I'd gone to great lengths to have another made, inscribed with our wedding date, and had surprised him with it during our wedding ceremony. I'd never really expected him to wear it, but from that day forward, he'd never taken it off.

I was happy that the ring meant so much to him and made no further reference to cancer or its potential doom that day. Smiling, I laid my head against the seat and rolled the window down, inviting the hot air to caress my face. I was glad that the weather in Michigan was unusually hot and dry that summer. Similar to Florida's, I was grateful for any reminder of where I wanted to be.

In the latter part of July, during the second week of the three-week chemo cycle, Neulasta, a once-a-week version of Neupogen, would stabilize my neutrophils, this time administered by our friend Jeff, a family physician. He was kind enough not to laugh at us either. I think Alex was still embarrassed about not giving me the shots himself, but everyone who knew of his reluctance tried hard to reassure him that he had nothing to be embarrassed about. Eventually, he even learned to laugh at himself about it.

That same week, I looked forward to spending an evening with three couples who wanted to visit. They didn't want to tire me, so they had volunteered to bring dinner. As we were setting the food out buffet style, my friend Oksana asked how I was doing. "Fine," I answered.

"But how are you really doing?" she pressed. "I mean,

are you coping okay?"

"I suppose I am," I answered.

"How about losing your hair? Has it been hard for you?"

"Well," I began, "I don't like losing my hair, but there are bigger fish to fry at the moment. I think the hardest thing about it is that it reminds me of my illness and makes me feel different. If I just *looked* like everybody else, then maybe I could *feel* like everybody else—healthy."

Oksana then asked, "May I go upstairs for a minute?" It sounded like an odd response, but I said, "Of course."

In minutes, she returned with my hats and scarves and began to hand them out to everyone. Alex chose the wide-brimmed, purple straw hat. Pavlo selected a pink scarf. And so it went, amidst much laughter, until all heads were covered. Oksana then turned to me and said, "Now we're all alike." Everyone kept their hats on for the duration of the evening, and I couldn't help but giggle at this motley hat brigade. Their antics were not only amusing, but they also showed so much love and support.

Throughout the summer, and in fact throughout my illness, I was very grateful that friends and acquaintances kept in touch. Sometimes I was just too tired to talk, but a message on the answering machine meant that someone cared. Cards, phone calls, and emails were humbling reminders that I mattered enough for others to take the time to contact me. It really never mattered what they said, but given my state of mind, I sometimes interpreted words differently than the way they were intended. For example, nearly everyone told me that my great attitude was sure to pull me through. I did have a good attitude most of the time, but did that mean it was my fault if I didn't make it? I loved the line that said, "Oh, you'll be just fine." Sometimes I wanted to reply, "Do you know something I don't?" One woman told me, "Hang in there. And just remember— where there's a will, there's a way." I really wanted to retort, "Listen, honey, I've got the will. Dr. Kaminski has the way. But don't blame either of us if I croak." And when anyone said, "I know how you feel," I wanted to scream back, "How could you?" Even an innocent and well-meaning statement of empathy like "I'm really worried about you," meant that I had the additional responsibility of cheering up yet one more person.

The line that seemed the most fraudulent of all was "You're facing this with such courage." I always wanted to set that record straight by answering, "No, I don't have one ounce of courage. I've never done a brave thing in my life. If I'd volunteered to have lymphoma for Juli or for Alex, that would have been brave. To tell you the truth, I'd rather be sucking my thumb."

And I hated it when people thought lymphoma was a virus. Although I'd only heard of the disease in recent years—and then only by chance—I was annoyed that everyone seemed to know about all types of cancer except those which were unattached to the word. I'd learned that, collectively, blood cancers were the third leading cause of death among the cancers, and that the incidence of lymphoma had doubled since the seventies, a fact which baffled scientists. And I would bitterly complain to Alex that public awareness of these facts must be raised. He would then challenge me to get well and do something about it, as if I could.

The words I treasured most were honest ones. When I looked terrible, "Hey, I like your blouse" was far more sincere than trying to convince me that I looked great. When I felt terrible, I appreciated a friend commiserating, "What a lousy thing you're going through," instead of trying to assure me that I was going to be just fine.

When a couple of friends sent books that had nothing to do with cancer, I valued their gestures as vivid demonstrations that they remembered me sans lymphoma. And when my dentist and his family sent a basket of beautifully decorated cookies, I was touched that they would remember me—and rather amused. "Doc, all that sugar. You looking for job security?" I teased.

If I twisted the intention of some remarks, it was only because my own confidence was shaken. Most people were truly wonderful, but I became a pariah to a few others. In mid-July, I ran into one of our former clients who nervously apologized for not calling after he had heard the news some months earlier. As an explanation, he offered, "I just can't handle illness. It makes me think I'll die." I almost laughed and asked, "So what makes you think you won't?" At least he was honest about it. Strangely, I heard from people from whom I would never have expected to hear and got the silent treatment from a few folks I thought would have called.

One wish that remained unfulfilled during my entire

illness was that someone—anyone—would send a card to Alex and Alex only. Everyone focused on me, and yet he had the much more difficult task of juggling work while trying to cope, often helplessly and always without training, with the ramifications of my illness. While people always asked about me when they saw him, no one ever actually took the time to write him a special note, a gesture that would have meant the world to me.

He was, after all, going through hell. Not only was he playing head cheerleader, he would also start dinner when he came home and found me asleep. He would vacuum when I was too tired. And he had already taken on much of my job. In addition to all that—and the normal daily challenges of building homes and preplanning the Mystic Ridge development—we had two of the most demanding situations we'd had in our careers. As the saying goes, when it rains, it pours.

One of these challenging situations had begun the previous December. We had just dug the hole for the foundation of a home when our clients decided to divorce. Lest building a home take the blame, it was the direct result of a cheatin' heart—which apparently wasn't the only cheating body part. We were peripherally drawn into the fray when Mr. and Mrs. Divorce stopped making payments on their construction loan. Consequently, we stopped getting paid, a small detail from which Alex protected me for several months. Out of the goodness of my heart, I offered to help them sell the house—free of charge—only to have Mr. Divorce, himself a cancer survivor, tell me quite emphatically and quite rudely that he didn't think I could handle it. I was devastated, but we ultimately did sell the house for them, although it was neither pleasant nor particularly profitable.

The other situation involved a couple for whom we had started construction shortly before I started chemo. It was clear from the beginning of the contract process that they were going to be difficult, and I bowed out, leaving Alex to work with them once chemo treatments began. Because this couple could not or would not make decisions about anything in a timely manner, how could we possibly order shingles without knowing which color they wanted or cabinets without knowing the doorstyle and finish? Nonetheless, they blamed Alex when construction fell behind schedule, and even he could not make them understand their role in the process or that their cooperation was crucial. Additionally, changes were made to changes, sometimes after items were installed. They also wanted all sorts of items at no cost and often tried to get them included through various and sundry sneaky and untruthful methods. A couple of costly items did slip through the cracks, and I asked Alex, after he had finally finished the house late in the year, why he had let that happen. He sighed deeply, his shoulders sagged, and he looked so weary that I thought he was going to cry when he answered, "Betsy, this year has been hell. How many battles can I fight?" I felt horrible.

Fortunately, our other clients couldn't have been more cooperative. They went out of their way to make choices on time and sometimes rescheduled their own busy lives so that our meetings were convenient for Alex and me. Months later, when I lightly and apologetically made fun of my chemo brain, all were surprised that I even had it. At first I thought I had concealed it better than I had remembered, but when I reviewed my journal as well as my files, I realized that Alex had almost always been around for every meeting I had.

During the summer, I gradually became very selective about which newspaper articles I read and which news shows I watched. Alex and I were accustomed to turning on TV news shows almost every evening. Even if we were doing something else, the news was always there in the background. But the horrors of one group slaying another seemed to dominate the news, and fighting for my own life, I was distressed by any unnecessary death and confounded by anyone who would sacrifice life for political ideology or any other reason.

Instead of the news, I watched funny movies and reruns of *I Love Lucy* and *M*A*S*H* or anything else that would buffer the grim reality of worldly conflicts or my lymphoma. I searched for stories about long shot victories. They were inspirational and reassuring as I dreamed of a victory of my own. And if I missed news about interest rates, I rationalized that somebody would fill me in.

In early August, a downtown theater was showing *Sunshine State*, an offbeat comedy about out-of-state developers trying to buy a small Florida town. I'd seen enough developers try to buy chunks of Florida to know that I would love the movie, but Alex and I were concerned about going to a public place where some stranger might sneeze. We decided we'd go during the week when fewer people might infect me. I could hardly wait for our date.

As we walked into the theater, I headed straight for the concession stand for popcorn and a Coke. Alex, always my great protector, gently suggested, "Betsy, we may be pushing it already. Don't you think you should skip this?"

"Absolutely not," I replied. "When's the last time we went out? Let's have a little fun."

Alex reminded me that we could have lots of fun without popcorn which may contain germs that could hurt me. "Why don't you just have the Coke?" he asked.

"My dear," I laughed, "I feel like being very naughty. Oooooooo—we're out in a public place. I'm about to have popcorn smothered in butter. And if you're a good boy, I'll share it with you." Alex knew then that the popcorn was non-negotiable, so he simply smiled, shook his head, and kissed my cheek.

For two hours during that movie, I felt like a normal human being. We enjoyed every morsel of popcorn and laughed at the one-liners about developers who tried, unsuccessfully, to gobble up more Florida real estate. We were still laughing as we walked arm-in-arm to the car. In the parking garage, I skipped circles around Alex, wanting the evening to last forever. It was the highlight of my entire summer.

Chemo brain had kept me mostly in oblivion during the summer. Days often passed without my knowing—or caring—whether it was Tuesday or Friday. I knew Sundays, though, because Ted and Lisa always brought dinner so that we wouldn't have to cook, and Greta and Zan usually joined us. It was the one routine that remained stable.

Frankly, I'm uncertain how I spent most days. I was somewhat frustrated that I couldn't garden. Spores in the dirt could cause infection. And though I had always been an avid reader, there were days when I was too tired to hold even a paperback. Anyway, reading sent me to slumberland after a few pages. I know that I spent many hours successfully teaching my constant companion, Tooties, to play catch. It was an activity which at least kept me awake and entertained, but which was hardly challenging. I was also thankful that I had never, not once, felt nauseated. And I marveled at other patients who said they were energized by chemotherapy and who seemed to be living their lives far more normally than I.

Mostly, my mind and body just seemed to be idling that summer. Some days were good. Some were bad. Sometimes I needed to talk about my illness. Sometimes I didn't. Most of the time, I didn't know what I wanted. How then could anyone else?

At least the drugs were winning the battle against the Invisible Invader, and Alex and I were happy that Neupogen, Neulasta, and my monumental cleanliness campaign had kept me out of Hotel Hell. And then, on Saturday morning, August 10, two days before the sixth treatment was scheduled, I awoke with a fever. Could there really have been germs in that popcorn—or had the Invisible Invader returned?

CHAPTER TEN

THE INVISIBLE INVADER
SCORES AGAIN

I wanted to ignore this latest incendiary, and if I couldn't ignore it, then I hoped that Dr. Kaminski would give me one of those little white slips of paper with indecipherable writing which would guarantee that I would quickly get well, otherwise known as a prescription. By late afternoon, when hot flashes raced through my body and clear visions of my father popped into my head without warning, I knew that no simple prescription would banish this ailment. The Invisible Invader was back, raging furiously. Several times I blinked back tears, not knowing how to break this news to Alex. What in the world were we going to do? I had been improving, and we were happy. Why was this happening? How much more could he take? How much more could I?

That night, I again dreamed about Daddy. I awoke from one dream only to fall back asleep and see his face again. This time he was silent, but I feared that I was in grave danger of joining him.

By morning, I was angry. This simply could not happen again. If I ignored the fever, it would disappear on its own. I was sure of it. I just had to do something *normal*. Before eight AM on that Sunday morning, I dragged out the vacuum cleaner and with gritted teeth and a fever of 101, I vacuumed the house as if to suck up every danger that surrounded me. Perplexed, Alex stood and watched. Afraid of crying, I couldn't look at him. Real normal, huh?

Alex wandered into our bedroom, where I finally turned off the vacuum, and asked if I was feeling okay. "I'm just fine," I announced defiantly through my still-gritted teeth. And with that I burst into tears, jumped back into our unmade bed, and pulled the covers over my head, hoping to find safety from fever and cancer and even death. Alex never did know what to do when I cried, but this time he sat on the edge of our bed and slowly pulled the covers from my head.

"What's going on?" he asked. I was sobbing so hard that I could barely tell him that the fever was back, my father wouldn't leave me alone, and I was sure the Invisible Invader was attacking again.

"I-I-I-I'm a-a-a-afraid I-I-I-I'm g-g-g-gonna d-d-d-die," I wailed.

Ever positive, Alex did his best to remind me that the recent CT scan had shown that chemo was doing its job. My father was just trying to let me know that he'll always watch over me. And the fever? The books, and Dr. Kaminski, said that fever could occur for many reasons. Wasn't I getting myself too worked up when there could be other explanations? No, I wasn't. I knew exactly what was going on inside my body, and I was filled with terror.

Alex tried so hard and so gently to comfort me, to convince me to keep my mind open to other explanations, and to keep hope alive. But no matter what he said, I could only sob deep, sorrowful, body-shaking sobs, and all Alex could do was stroke my head and hand me tissues. Lots of tissues.

When I finally lifted my head off my waterlogged pillow, we decided to call the hospital. Within minutes, Dr. Kaminski returned the call and, like Alex, assured me that there could be many explanations. Since I was scheduled to see him the following morning prior to the next chemo treatment, he suggested that we wait until morning to do anything, unless the fever increased, and then I was to head to the emergency room. Dr. Kaminski always had a soothing effect on me, and I was willing to hope that this was anything but another attack of the Invisible Invader. So was Alex.

But hope was one thing. Reality was another, and I could not ignore the symptoms that were threatening my life. In my angst, I decided that I could at least make life easier for Alex and Juli after I was gone. I would sort through some family items, mark them well, and set them aside. I began with some jewelry that had belonged to my grandmothers. I placed the pieces in small boxes and identified the original owners, not sure if Juli would remember. I placed the boxes in Ziploc bags and put them in one of my dresser drawers. And then I showed Alex what I had accomplished and asked him please to give the bags to Juli when I was dead and gone.

Horrified, he asked, "Betsy, what are you doing this for?"

"I just thought it would make it easier for everybody," I answered matter-of-factly. Alex pulled me close to him and begged me to think of living, not dying. And just how was I supposed to ignore that distinct possibility with fevers and hot flashes raging again?

By late afternoon, the fever had spiked to 103. Following Dr. Kaminski's instructions, Alex and I headed for the emergency room. Our hope was renewed when the emergency room doctor checked for pneumonia. Alex and I were actually *happy* to hear pneumonia, and I scoffed, "What's wrong with this picture? We're glad I might have pneumonia?" We chuckled at how our perspectives had changed during the year. We didn't chuckle when the X-ray was clear. The doctor sent us home to await our appointment with Dr. Kaminski the following morning.

In the emergency room, my hopes lifted. Maybe I *was* overreacting to this fever. Perhaps I was plain paranoid. But by the time we arrived home, close to midnight, I was convinced that the disease had returned. The symptoms were all too familiar, and that's exactly what I told Dr. Kaminski and Judy the following morning, much to Alex's chagrin. There I was, losing hope again, he feared.

Always the optimist, Dr. Kaminski tried to reassure us that we couldn't be certain without scientific data, but I was sure I saw worry in his and Judy's eyes, and I made some sarcastic remark like, "You can gather all the scientific data you want. You and I both know it's back." Graciously ignoring my sarcasm, he said we would have some tests and make a determination when we had the results. And he reminded me that we still had options. There were other chemotherapies, radioimmunotherapy, and, just in case, we should type Karen's and my blood to learn if she would be a suitable donor if we needed a bone marrow transplant.

A bone marrow transplant? I wasn't ready to think about that, much less discuss it. At our first meeting with Dr. Kaminski, I recalled that a bone marrow transplant was the last treatment he mentioned. While he had thoroughly explained all the others, he had said that he didn't want to go into the details of a transplant at that time, adding that it was the last option. I also knew that a transplant was risky. Now, seven months later, that last option was reintroduced as a possibility. Dr. Kaminski sensed my panic, assured me that we simply needed to be ready if necessary, and reminded me that we had a long way to go before a transplant.

I loved the way Dr. Kaminski and Judy—and in fact all their colleagues—said *we*. Sometimes it almost made me laugh, like when they said, "*We* will have a CT scan." I came close to asking if they meant we'd have a group picture, all of us lying together on the narrow slab and sliding through the machine. Humor aside, their choice of this simple, small word implied that they respected my feelings. *We* indicated to me that they were treating me as their partner, when in fact I always saw Dr. Kaminski as the commander-in-chief, Judy as his adjutant, and myself as merely an unwilling draftee.

We did not have chemotherapy that day. Instead, Dr. Kaminski prescribed Decadron, a steroid which reduces fever, can kill malignant lymphocytes, and causes insomnia. Decadron was a stopgap measure until *we* determined the future course of action, which would depend on the results of another CT scan and bone marrow biopsy, both scheduled for the following day.

Once again, Carolyn Shearer would perform the biopsy. By now, her friendly manner had made me feel very comfortable with her, even though she still wielded her jackhammer. However, experience had proven that Versed would eliminate any pain, and so I no longer dreaded the procedure. I should have. Or I should have taken more Versed. This time, I remembered every single tap-tap-tap of that needle, and it hurt. I liked the noninvasive CT scan much better. Somebody simply pressed a button in another room and knew immediately what was happening inside. No muss. No fuss. No needles.

Still feeling the effect of Versed, I went to sleep early that evening. Juli, calling to find out how I felt, spoke with Alex. Later I would learn that he told her we were running out of options. She promised to find a way to come up to see me, a big step for someone who absolutely hates to fly. I'd planned to fly down the second I finished chemo, but this new development made my travel plans very uncertain.

Wednesday morning arrived, and leaving "our" options to Dr. Kaminski, I considered what I was to do. Since my body seemed so determined to kill me, it occurred to me that I should write my own obituary. Left to Alex, he might simply say, "Betsy died." Oh, how very eloquent. But how does one write one's own obituary without sounding pompous? I abandoned the idea. Should I at least plan a funeral? Choose the music? I smirked as I thought that "Stayin' Alive" would be a little late, not to mention inappropriate. And just why was I dwelling on my own demise? I was thrilled that my daughter and grandbabies were coming, and surely Dr. Kaminski would come up with something.

Later in the day, he called with the test results. His scientific data proved what I already knew. The score was 2–0, the Invisible Invader over Betsy. I had failed CVP and I had failed CHOP with Rituxan. Or did they fail me? What now? What was the back up plan?

"Betsy, I've made all the arrangements for you to take Zevalin. You'll have to go to another clinic because we're not set up to give it. I've already talked to the doctors there and you have an appointment next Monday." Whoa, Dr. Kaminski. You did what? You transferred me and my cancer cells to another hospital? To take Zevalin? Your very own Bexxar's rival?

I asked Dr. Kaminski if I would be his first patient to take Zevalin. When he answered yes, I couldn't help but say, "Oh, Dr. Kaminski, thank you, but I'm so sorry. You must have taken a little heat from the doctors over there."

Half chuckling, he answered, "Yes, I took a little ribbing, but this is the best thing we can do for you right now."

I knew about Zevalin. It was a type of radioimmunotherapy (RIT) and was the direct competitor of Dr. Kaminski's Bexxar, the drug he had spent years developing and which was still under FDA review. As I understood it, radioimmunotherapy grew from the idea of treating cancer with antibodies, a theory that dates back to 1908 when German bacteriologist Paul Erlich won a Nobel Prize for his studies of the immune system. Erlich believed that it might be possible to attach substances to antibodies which would then kill tumors without harming normal cells. However, scientists were unable to perfect Erlich's theory because they could not produce pure lines of antibodies which would target cancerous cells.

It wasn't until 1972 that German immunologists discovered how to produce pure lines of antibodies, called monoclonal antibodies. Researchers at first believed that these antibodies might be able to kill cancerous cells without attaching additional substances to them. However, the antibodies needed a target on tumor cells which they could recognize and to which they could attach. Unfortunately, no one could find a target that appeared only on tumor cells. By the mid-eighties, most scientists had given up.

Not Dr. Kaminski. He and his U of M colleague, Dr. Richard Wahl, doggedly continued to search for answers, and their persistence paid off. They developed a treatment, Bexxar, using CD20 antibodies, found on the surface of all B-cell lymphomas, and they tagged it with radioactive iodine which delivers radiation to tumor cells. In effect, they created a guided missile. The antibody seeks, finds, and attaches itself to the protein found on the surface of lymphoma cells, and the radioactive substance destroys them.

In 1990, Dr. Kaminski began testing his theory on

patients with remarkable results. In the medical world, news like this travels fast. Another drug company later began work on its own version of this radiolabeled antibody, and they called it Zevalin. In a neck-and-neck race to bring the two drugs to market, Zevalin received accelerated approval by the FDA in February 2002. The approval was based on studies of 197 patients. I didn't get it. Bexxar had been studied on more patients—and longer.

I had been closely watching this race and had hoped that Bexxar would be approved in case I needed it. Why couldn't the Invisible Invader have waited to return until after Bexxar's approval? I was, after all, Dr. Kaminski's patient, and if I needed RIT, I certainly wanted to take his drug, but that was impossible. All the Bexxar clinical trials which would fit my situation were closed.

Zevalin was my only option, but I couldn't understand why the FDA approved it based on shorter studies and fewer patients than Bexxar. From my perspective, it was scary to think that the FDA would approve any drug based on studies of just 197 patients, and I couldn't help but think that money and politics had won that bureaucratic race.

Once again, Dr. Kaminski came to my rescue. As a leading expert on radioimmunotherapy, and thoroughly familiar with the differences between Bexxar and Zevalin, he was confident that Zevalin was a reasonable choice. And I was confident in him.

After Dr. Kaminski and I said goodbye, I sat at my desk, pondering this development. It was certainly wonderful that I could have cutting edge treatment, but Dr. Kaminski had spent his career developing a drug to save lymphoma patients, and together with his colleagues, had fought every battle with me. If I was going to be anyone's success, I was going to be his. No one else's. Period.

I called Alex and shared the news with him. He was so thankful that Dr. Kaminski had made all the necessary arrangements—and so quickly. When I told him I'd wait for Bexxar's approval because I wanted to be Dr. Kaminski's success, Alex immediately saw the bigger picture. "How could you possibly be his success if you refuse the very drug that may save your life?"

After continuing to resist for awhile longer, I finally saw the light. "Okay, so I was just having a blond moment," I quipped.

"No excuses. You don't have any blond anymore," Alex teased, no doubt breathing a sigh of relief. I laughed and suddenly realized that Dr. Kaminski clearly didn't care who got the credit for getting me well. His ego never came into play. My wellness was his only concern. And my respect for him turned to awe.

But I would have to leave him and his colleagues to take Zevalin. Believing that Bexxar's approval was imminent, U of M had not arranged to administer Zevalin. I'd have to go to another hospital and another hematology clinic. Dread stabbed at me. All my old fears about the health care system resurfaced. There would be a whole new group of people who would be clueless about me and my life, and now more than ever I needed the familiarity of the people I knew and trusted.

"I *hate* the FDA for expelling me from my own U of M sanctuary," I whined to Alex. "What's wrong with those people?"

Alex would have preferred to stay at U of M as well, but always more rational than I, he saw that it wasn't an option. Reminding me of the success of radioimmunotherapy, he would say, "Try to forget about everything else and focus on the outcome." Easy for you to say, I thought.

At the end of that week, Judy called to ask how I was feeling, and I told her I was feeling fine. The real reason for her call was to assure me that she and Dr. Kaminski were not abandoning me. "We'll always be here for you," she said so sweetly that I almost cried. Her call was one of many that buoyed my spirits throughout my illness.

Later in the day, I told Alex about Judy's call. "She's not just a nurse. She's a saint," I said, "*and* chief angel on this earth. Every doctor should have a Judy." Alex agreed, thinking to himself that every kindness she—or anyone—had extended to me had also given him a brief reprieve from playing head cheerleader.

On Monday, August 20, Alex took me and my cancer cells to the new hematology clinic. The new doctor talked about refractory lymphoma and Zevalin. He reminded us that chemo-resistant lymphoma is not a good sign. Great, tell us something we don't know. By now, he said, Zevalin had been administered to about eight hundred, maybe one thousand patients, and it was so new that there were simply no studies available to indicate its long-term effectiveness, especially on patients who had failed chemo. I wanted to scream back, "I didn't fail chemo. It failed me." Then he added that I'd be lucky for it to hold my lymphoma in check for ten months. He suggested that I talk with the bone marrow transplant unit at U of M as soon as possible.

Although this new doctor was nice enough, his words and his body language clearly conveyed, "There's not a lot of hope for you." Fragile as I was, this message only magnified my fears and frustrations. Looking back, he didn't listen to his own words: *no studies are available to indicate its long-term effectiveness.* That was a fact, and there is where he should have stopped. Adding that I might be dead in ten months, Dr. Doom dampened every hope I had.

Walking to the car after our meeting, I once again buried my head in Alex's shoulder and sobbed. "Ten months? Why bother? And then what? A bone marrow transplant? You mean the same thing that killed King Hussein? No thanks. I won't do it."

Alex stopped walking, put one hand on each of my shoulders, turned to me, and said, with as much authority in his voice as he could muster, "Betsy, remember that Dr. Kaminski has been studying these drugs for years. He's a scientist, a researcher, as well as a physician. No wonder he's comfortable with them. You can't let a few comments get you down."

Hearing little, my eyes widened as they always do when I try to make a point, and I replied sadly, "Alex, if you think ten days in the hospital was hard, you ain't seen nothin'. I've read a little about transplants and I don't want to put you—

or me—through it. I can't. It's that simple." My chin was quivering hard when I looked straight into his eyes and added, "If all I have left is a few months, then can't we just make the most of them without a bunch of horrible treatments? Can't we just go off and be happy?"

There in the parking lot, Alex threw his head back and sighed, not knowing what else to say. He drew me close to him, held me tenderly, and ran one hand through the faux fur. Chuckling through my tears, I whimpered, "Don't even *think* about pulling my wig off."

Drawing me even closer, he gently whispered back, "I promise I won't if you'll promise to keep all your options open."

With our arms still around each other, I pushed away from his shoulder, looked straight at him, and smirked, "I'd rather you pull the wig off."

"*Bet-sy*," he countered authoritatively, peering over his glasses.

"Okay, you win. I'll keep my options open."

It was already late afternoon by the time we headed home. The support group was meeting that night, and I had planned to go. I hadn't missed a meeting since I'd first attended, but I just couldn't muster the happy face that I felt I needed to wear. In fact, I was afraid that I would melt into tears, and since I'd never seen anyone break down at a meeting, I wasn't about to be the first.

But there was another reason I didn't go. I didn't want to leave Alex. Not only did I need to be near him, but I also knew that I had upset him that afternoon. I thought that if

I cooked dinner and talked about work, he would believe I'd just had a little outburst and had gotten over it. He didn't believe it. He would tell me later that he was just as scared as I was. Scared of that new door that had opened. Scared that I wouldn't pass through it, even if it became my only option. And scared that neither of us was up to that challenge. It would require enormous energy to push thoughts of a transplant aside while we focused on the Zevalin treatment.

But obtaining this new drug would not be an easy task. Zevalin is not stocked on the shelves of drugstores. Each dose is made to order and sent to the facility where it is administered. And although it had been approved by the FDA, insurance companies had not yet approved payment for it, and it would take Herculean efforts to persuade our insurance carrier to cover this expensive drug. I knew none of this at the time, but the facts began to unfold over the next several days as it became clear that, among other things, Dr. Kaminski had to write a letter of medical need. In other words, some bean counter was about to decide whether I could have this life-saving drug or not.

Carolyn became my new best friend. She protected me from the details as much as possible, reminding me that I had enough stress without this additional worry. She promised to do what was necessary to make sure that insurance covered the treatment, and I believed her. No one at U of M had ever let me down yet. She'll never admit to the hours she spent wrangling with the insurance company, but she prevailed, and we will be forever grateful. We'd have been in big trouble otherwise.

I began to feel like a zombie that week. Decadron had kicked in, and I was sleeping very little. And still manipulating my mind, chemo brain remembered the last thing it heard, which was that I had ten months to live—if, of course, I was lucky. Exhausted and plagued by relapse, I could barely think. I neither laughed nor cried. I simply existed, waiting and wondering if Zevalin would work—and for how long.

I no longer hoped to see my grandchildren graduate from college. Seeing them start kindergarten seemed a stretch. I'd wanted a new winter coat, but how many winters would I get out of it? I stopped thinking about a new coat. The newspaper subscription was due for renewal. I had a choice of paying for three months, six months, or a year. I paid for three months and wondered if that was too long. And more pieces of my life fell victim to the Invisible Invader when I resigned that week from every committee I sat on.

By the weekend, while Alex and I were straightening the garage and I was thinking about the past few cancerous months and the dilemma in which we now found ourselves, I happened to notice his wading boots hanging from a hook. I looked at those big heavy wading boots and laughed out loud. "What's funny?" Alex asked.

"You see those wading boots?"

"Yeah," he replied quizzically.

Chuckling, I told him I wanted to make a videotape for Dr. Kaminski and Judy and Carolyn and all the others who had worked on my case. I would wear his wading boots, symbolic of wading through cancer, treatments, side effects, etc. Then I would fill a bucket with different kinds of balls, each one representing the different treatments. Next I would throw each ball at the basketball hoop, only to miss the basket as far as chemo missed its mark. At the end of the tape, I would look straight into the camera and say, "Thanks to the excellent treatments available for lymphoma, I still play basketball as well as I did before I took them."

By the time I finished spinning this preposterous tale, I was laughing uproariously. Incredulous, Alex had cocked his eyebrows straight up and hadn't even cracked a smile. Looking at him made me laugh even harder. "Come on, Alex, don't you think that's even a little funny? Can't you just picture playing that tape for all the doctors when they meet to discuss patients?"

Shaking his head, he replied, "I think they'd forget about treating lymphoma and send you straight to Tom," meaning our friend Tom Fluent, the psychiatrist.

"Oh, that's perfect," I laughed. "A straightjacket to go with the waders." Even my sense of humor had warped.

Early the following week, I had to see yet another stranger, the radiation oncologist who would actually pump me full of Zevalin. Although he would be my personal cellular executioner, I dreaded going to another doctor. I shouldn't have. Dr. Jafar would have made a wonderful coach. He examined the playing field—me—and with the greatest of confidence, explained the defensive play— Zevalin. And then he wheeled around on his stool, took a deep breath, placed both hands on his knees, and began to deliver the best pep talk I've ever had.

"Look," he said. "Until they've been around for awhile, there is a lot we don't know about new drugs. But what we do know is that Zevalin can work for you." Little could he have known that I was sitting on the table thinking, "Yeah, for ten months."

Dr. Jafar continued, and passionately. "You know, Betsy," yes, he actually used my name, "I've been a physician for a long time. I've seen people live who shouldn't have, medically speaking. I've seen people die who, medically, should have lived. Sometimes there is no reason for either outcome. What I've observed over the years is that the people who fight back, whose will to live is the strongest, who maintain positive outlooks, they're most often the ones who beat the odds. I will give you the best medicine that is currently available, but you have a job to do, too. You go home and you fight. Eat right. Get plenty of rest. Love your family. Laugh often. And don't give up—not for a minute."

I sat on the table listening to this speech, speechless. There was a doctor telling me I had a chance! My eyes grew a little misty and my spirit soared. Maybe I could make it for eleven months, even twelve? Did I dare hope for longer? I would gladly follow Dr. Jafar's instructions if that meant boosting my chance for success, but did ten minutes of sleep a week qualify as plenty of rest? Decadron wasn't allowing much more.

My outlook began to lift as Labor Day weekend and the arrival of Juli and the babies approached. A full eight

months had passed since I had seen them, and just imagining holding those babies put a smile on my face. I didn't
want to miss one waking moment of their visit, but I was
somewhat concerned that I would not be able to match their
energy levels. Two days before their arrival, I was happily
buying bubbles and baby food and never gave a second
thought to the blood test I had that morning.

On Thursday, exactly one hour before leaving to meet
Juli, Skye, and Nicholas at the airport, I was jittery with
euphoric anticipation when the phone rang. It was the
doctor at the new hematology clinic. The blood test from
two days earlier indicated that my lymphocyte count had
soared to twenty, twice the high end of the range in which
Zevalin could safely be administered. Although the test dose
was scheduled for the following Wednesday, it was doubtful,
he said, that I was a candidate for Zevalin. He asked me to
have a blood test the following Tuesday, and then we said
goodbye.

I wanted to clinch my fists and scream. I wanted to
throw things. I wanted to hit something. I wanted to scream
louder and harder. But as usual, I turned to Alex, who thankfully happened to be home working, and sobbed uncontrol-
lably on his shoulder. My body tensed as it had never done
before, and after sobbing for several minutes, I think it
would have collapsed into a heap on the floor had Alex not
supported it in his arms. A second relapse and now this?
Oh, dear God. What did it mean if I couldn't take Zevalin?
What would stop this monstrous Invisible Invader that
seemed so determined to murder me? Was there any bottom

to this emotional abyss?

And just why had Dr. Doom waited two whole days to call me? The results of blood tests can be reported in minutes, not days. It was *my* blood and I had a right to know quickly when it misbehaved. Yeah, I wanted to shoot the messenger. His delivery was terrible. His timing was worse. Had he called even an hour earlier, we might have had the time to find out if other options were available prior to the dreaded bone marrow transplant—if a suitable donor could even be found in a short time. But there was no time for that now. Juli and her babies were somewhere over Ohio and approaching Detroit fast. I wasn't even sure I could stop the flow of tears, much less manage a smile when they arrived.

I dragged myself upstairs to wash my face and to change the shirt onto which mascara-stained tears had fallen. I left Alex downstairs, standing in the kitchen, arms by his sides. His shoulders drooped, his eyebrows were drawn together, his color drained. He looked so weary. When I returned downstairs, he hadn't moved. He wanted to drive me to the airport, but luggage and carseats left little room for another passenger. I promised him I was okay, at least to drive, and we melted together in a long embrace. As I opened the door to the garage, I turned my head over my shoulder and practiced smiling. "You might want to change your shirt. My mascara's not your color." He didn't smile back.

In the car, I desperately wanted to call *somebody* to help me cope with this maelstrom. What were our options? Did we have any left? Was I facing a transplant in thirty days?

Sixty? What if Karen didn't match? Would anyone? What if no one did? And why had Dr. Doom delivered such awful news without suggesting an alternative plan or at least giving me some form of reassurance? Didn't he have a clue that news like this would devastate anybody?

Dr. Kaminski and Judy were on vacation. I thought of calling Carolyn, but I was well aware that I would have started bawling again if I even heard her voice. I *couldn't* call her then. My puffy eyes and red nose from the last cry needed the drive time to recover before I met Juli. Alex was too numb to think of calling Carolyn for me, and I was too numb to think of asking him. Somehow I *had* to pull myself together, to draw on my own reserves. I hoped I had some left.

CHAPTER ELEVEN

BELIEVE IN MIRACLES

Fighting tears and pounding my fists on the steering wheel during the forty-five-minute drive to the airport, I pulled into the parking garage, wiped my eyes dry, and hoped they would stay that way. Waiting for Juli, Nicholas, and Skye at the baggage claim area, I wondered how the kids would react to me. Nicholas, at eighteen months, hadn't even been walking when I saw him last. He couldn't possibly remember me. I knew that Skye, who had just turned three, would.

My heart raced with excitement when I saw them in the distance. Spotting me, Skye pulled away from Juli and ran with outstretched arms, knocking me off my knees as I knelt to catch her. At last her little arms were around my neck and I smothered her with kisses. "Grammy, Grammy, I love you," she said. Her exuberance immediately banished my anguish to the farthest recesses of my mind. And at last I embraced Juli, the daughter I had missed so terribly all year. Nicholas, though smiling, wasn't sure who I was. We would have to get to know each other again.

Surrounded by the three people I had missed the most, we headed home to play for the next four days. Throwing caution to the wind, I ventured out into the germ-infested world, determined to enjoy Juli and my grandchildren. Did anybody know when—or if—I could do it again? We played on swings and slides. We spent a day at the Toledo Zoo. Even Juli cautioned me to remain outside the petting area, but I wasn't about to miss Skye's and Nicholas's giggles and squeals as they played with the baby animals. We toured the fire station and a hands-on museum for children.

Late Saturday afternoon, we visited a tiger exhibit and held baby tigers, much to the kids' delight. While there, Carolyn phoned to ask how I was feeling. "Fine," I assured her, without telling her what we were doing. I added, "Carolyn, it's Saturday afternoon. You must have better things to do than to call me. Go enjoy the rest of the weekend." In fact, Carolyn was not calling solely to inquire about how I felt. The real purpose of her call was to report that Karen's blood was incompatible with mine and to recommend that Juli's be typed. This was not good news, but at the moment, I was too busy with my grandbabies and the tigers to care.

At home, we filled the jacuzzi with bubbles and became bubble monsters, amidst uproarious laughter. We chased one another around the house playing hide and seek. Skye and I baked cakes and cookies.

Afraid that my mangy head might frighten the kids, I always wore a knit cap when I wasn't wearing the wig. One evening, before I could stop him, Nicholas pulled off the cap, and both he and Skye immediately froze, staring at my head. Finally, Skye asked, "Grammy, what happened to your hair?"

"I took some medicine that made it fall out," I answered.

"Oh, I not take that kind of medicine," she said, quickly resuming her laughter and nonstop chatter. Nicholas stroked my head as if it belonged to one of the baby goats at the zoo. And that was the end of that. Shouldn't I have known that kids accept far more than we adults realize?

For four days, uncertainty stayed in the background while we laughed and played and hugged and kissed. Despite the potential crisis that lay ahead, my energy level rose to its highest level of the year. Alex, on the other hand, was clearly distraught. He was pleasant enough but could scarcely manage a smile. His voice sounded flat and barely audible. His lifeless eyes seemed focused on something in the distance. His frequent hugs that weekend were powerful and poignant. Did I sense grief?

When Juli's visit came to an end, I was sad to see them go but glad that she and the babies had come. Every moment with them gave me a precious memory and plenty of reminders of why I should fight for life with every ounce of my strength. After returning them to the airport on Tuesday morning, I proceeded straight to the hospital for the blood test. What had my lymphocytes been doing all weekend while the rest of me played? Had those murderous little cells been multiplying wantonly?

My cell phone rang two hours after the blood test. Caller ID, indicating Dr. Doom, turned my stomach queasy. I barely managed to answer before voice mail picked up. "Hello," I said, trying to sound perfectly normal.

"Hello, Mrs. de Parry. I don't know how this happened, but your lymphocyte count dropped to two. Come on in tomorrow for the Zevalin." Astonished, I'm sure my voice quivered as I thanked him for calling.

Jumping up and down with tears of joy falling down my cheeks, I excitedly dialed Alex's phone. "It's a miracle. My lymphocytes are down to two!" And then I became Ethel Merman, bellowing out in song, "I got Zevalin. I got Zevalin. I got Zevalin. Who could ask for anything more?" Never mind that I have a range of one note, which is reliably flat—the song said it all. Delivered from whatever potential disaster might have awaited us had my lymphocyte count remained high, we were more excited than two kids on Christmas morning. And that night, resurrected from despair, we both badly sang Ethel's song with our own words as we danced around the kitchen. Okay, *I* danced around the kitchen. Alex is much too reserved for such silliness, but his broad smile was a perfectly suitable dance partner.

Skeptics may attribute the fall in my lymphocyte count to Decadron, but they'd certainly disregarded the drug the previous week. I believe the fall was the direct result of hundreds of baby kisses and all the love and happiness I experienced that weekend. Scientists can't explain it, but they do know that endorphins—those chemicals which control the body's reaction to pain and stress—can have a mighty impact on our immune systems, and I believe that my endorphins gobbled up those unruly lymphocytes, thanks to Juli and Nicholas and Skye and the miracle of love.

The following morning, we hauled me and my low

lymphocyte count to the other hospital. Preceded by an infusion of Rituxan, Zevalin is administered twice, one week apart. The first dose was a very small amount of the drug for imaging purposes. Scans on three subsequent days determined that the drug was settling and clearing properly. Thankfully, the scans indicated that the drug was behaving exactly as it should.

Alex and I celebrated our fourth anniversary that weekend. He had asked what I wanted and I had jokingly said, "Your karma. Or how about some new blood?" We made dinner at home and were happy to celebrate the day.

On Sunday, Alex asked if there was anything I would like to do that day. "Go to Hell," I deadpanned. His eyes widened questioningly. "I want to go to Hell." And so we did. Hell, Michigan, is a tiny little village approximately one half hour northwest of Ann Arbor. Mimicking the "Got Milk?" ad campaign, I made a "Got Lymphoma?" banner. In Hell, I placed it so that the entire sign read "Got Lymphoma? Welcome to Hell." Alex took pictures of me by the sign, and I emailed them to several friends who saw the humor in it far more than he did.

On Wednesday, September 11, the sun was just beginning to peer over the horizon when we left home and headed to the hospital for the full blast of Zevalin. Alex and I spoke of the date and grieved for the thousands of families whose loved ones had lost their lives one year earlier. Yet we were giddy with hope that the day would spring new life into me. Halfway to the hospital, the sun's rays were bathing the earth with radiant beams, and I broke into song, "Oh, what a beautiful morning. Oh, what a beautiful day. I've got a beautiful feeling. Everything's going our way." Alex smiled and patted my hand and failed to mention that my vocal chords needed tuning.

At the hematology clinic, we met with the doctor shortly before the infusion. Again he reminded us that there was no way of knowing how long Zevalin would contain the disease, six months maybe. Hadn't he said ten months at our earlier meeting? Don't steal four months from me now. I told him to quit worrying, that I would be around to change Alex's bedpan in our old age. I was so exuberant that nothing could dampen my mood.

Almost nothing. Moments before the Rituxan infusion began, a sharp pain suddenly stabbed at my right side. I joked to Alex, "Maybe I got too excited this morning. I think I'm having an anxiety attack." Except that it wasn't funny. I could barely breathe. The nurse checked with the doctor who ordered Motrin, and the infusion got underway.

This was the big moment. The end of treatment. The day the Invisible Invader would be slain and our lives could return to normal. I was sure of it. For Alex, I'd brought pom-poms and a card which thanked him for being my biggest cheerleader, and he laughed when I gave them to him. Mr. Reserved even waved the pom-poms and chanted, "Kill the cells. Kill the cells. Go Zevalin."

Four hours later, when the Rituxan infusion was complete and I was still in pain and breathing as shallowly as possible, the nurse again checked with the doctor. I guess I thought that he would walk across the hall and see me like

Judy had done when I'd had a reaction to the first Rituxan treatment. Instead, the nurse returned with additional Motrin and a bomb for a possible explanation for the pain. She reported matter-of-factly, "The doctor feels that the cancer has spread to your bone. Here's a prescription for pain." And then she left the room. Stunned, I looked at Alex and said, "Great, now we deal with bone cancer. That's nice and fatal."

Still slightly groggy from the Benadryl which I had taken before the Rituxan infusion, I didn't thoroughly absorb the explanation for my pain. Alex, however, was completely alert, and weeks later would tell me that he was enraged that a nurse had delivered such unhappy news—and on what basis? No X-ray, no CT scan, no other test had been taken on which to base that assumption. No doctor had examined me for this symptom. And no one made a single suggestion about what we should do if it were true, unless you count the prescription for painkillers. And if that was the best they could do for me, the outlook was indeed bleak. Every bit of Alex's optimism was massacred by that nurse's words. She'd no sooner said them than he immediately began to ponder how abruptly and drastically things can change and to wonder what horrors would be next.

Alex would also tell me later that I seemed to have forgotten the news quickly and was excitedly declaring, "By this time tomorrow, I'll be cancer-free." Thank goodness for Benadryl. Meanwhile, panicked and angry, he was struggling to appear calm. He wanted to leave the room and find a phone to call Judy or Dr. Kaminski, thinking that they had never, not once, dismissed any little ache or pain as too trivial to investigate prior to making assumptions, nor had they ever left us dangling with bad news without offering some reassurance to offset it. But Zevalin was on its way, and he remained by my side.

Save for Alex, the mood in my tiny room was festive, as if some spectacular event were about to take place. Radioactive fireworks, I thought. They didn't call this nuclear medicine for nothing. Since I was the third Zevalin recipient at this hospital, several doctors wanted to watch the show, and the star soon arrived neatly packed in a metal box bearing a radioactive label which I read to Alex as, "Danger. Touch this stuff and you die. Remember Chernobyl. Ah, that could be my new name. But you can call me Cherry— Cherry de Parry. Ha ha ha." Alex just rolled his eyes.

I then asked rhetorically, "Isn't it remarkable that radiation cures the same way it kills—by destroying cells? Thank God for all the scientists who made this moment possible." And whispering to Alex so the other doctors wouldn't hear, I added, "Especially Dr. Kaminski. This may not be his drug, but it's *his* theory." Squeezing my hand, he tried to smile. I remember wondering why he looked so anxious. Hadn't he been the one to encourage me to remain hopeful?

Within another half hour, Dr. Jafar and Zevalin had thoroughly bathed my cells with radioactive missiles, and it was time to go home. Exiting the hospital and delighting in the sun's warmth, I threw my hands in the air, danced in circles, and rejoiced. "Yea, I'm done. I'm down to one blood test a week. We have our lives back." Why did the look on

Alex's face seem to disagree with me? Because he knew better. He was simply too kind to remind me that my body was so toxified that it would need some recovery time. And there was that little bone cancer issue.

I was far more alert the following day. I still had pain and breathing was difficult. I remembered the cause was supposed to be bone cancer. I didn't fill the prescription for painkillers. And I didn't call Dr. Kaminski or Judy that day, nor would I let Alex. I begged him to give me one day—just one day—to believe that I was cancer-free before I faced any subsequent setbacks. And all day I hoped that the pain would magically disappear. It didn't.

With all the setbacks I'd had, I felt like a hypochondriac by the time I called Judy the following day. "Come on in to the clinic," she said. Alex said he would be right home to drive me, but suspecting that I would have tests during which he'd be sitting in waiting rooms, I suggested he stay at work. I'd call him, I promised.

In the form of scans and ultrasounds, Dr. Kaminski ordered so many different photographs of my interior that day that I was sure U of M would run out of film. By six PM, he suspected that a small blood clot was the possible culprit, a far superior explanation than bone cancer, I thought. He couldn't be certain without an angiogram, which, since it was Friday, could not be done until the following Monday unless he admitted me to the hospital. Another stay in Hotel Hell? I don't think so. Ever cautious, I knew that Dr. Kaminski would not let me return home if he believed I was in any danger. To be safe, he prescribed a blood thinner that I was to take over the weekend.

When Judy brought the prescription to me, I laughed at its label. "Dr. Kaminski, this must be a mistake. It's an aphrodisiac. It says Lovenox—love in the night. Alex will love it." He laughed and corrected my pronunciation of "love-nox" to "lov-eh-nox" with a long "o."

There was just one small problem with this aphrodisiac. It required self-injections—*twice* daily. I could find friends to administer shots once a day, but twice? Dr. Kaminski hadn't heard about Alex's and my cowardice before, and he chuckled when I told him Alex had once planned to become a surgeon. "Probably a good thing he chose another line of work," he said. Judy gave me the first shot that afternoon, and once again stayed well past clinic hours to assist with my care.

Alex and I were so relieved. Almost anything was better than bone cancer. By the time I arrived home, after seven, Alex had dinner ready and waiting, after which I announced, "We have a problem. I have to take shots twice a day. Who can I mooch off of this time?"

Slowly, Alex rose from the table, walked to the bar, and poured himself a glass of wine. And then he turned to me, grinned broadly, raised his glass, and said, "Here's to your new nurse. *I'll* give you the shots."

"Sure you will," I laughed. "You almost passed out when Sandy tried to hand you the syringe."

"I can do it," he tried to assure me. "I just need to psych myself up for it. I don't want to hurt you."

"Here's your big chance," I teased.

And how was Alex *not* going to hurt me, considering the fact that he had never held a syringe, much less emptied its contents into another human being? We got an orange and one of the used syringes from the Neupogen, and he practiced injecting the fruit over and over again.

By morning, when it was time for the next shot, I was certain that we'd be found passed out on the floor with a syringe dangling from my leg if we foolishly proceeded. Alex, on the other hand, was intent on accomplishing the mission. Nervous but determined, he practiced a few more times on the orange while I panicked and paced around the kitchen island muttering absurdities. "Oh God, it's Dr. Mengele reincarnated and experimenting again. Alex, no matter how badly you hurt me, I swear I'll still love you. Don't you want to rethink this? If you don't give me the shots and it *is* a blood clot, maybe it will hit my heart and we'll both be out of our misery."

"Will you just shut up?" he said, laughing at me. "I'm ready." The syringe he was holding straight in the air looked like a rifle, and I waited for someone to announce, "Ready. Aim. Fire." And then I'd be gone—after an agonizing bombardment, of course.

"Okay, let's get this over with," I whimpered.

I sat down, swabbed my leg with alcohol, and pinched my thigh for him. And then I closed my eyes and waited for unskilled hands to inflict grisly torture. The waiting was interminable. What was he doing? I moaned and moaned and moaned and finally begged through gritted teeth, "Alex, just push it in. I swear I won't scream, no matter how much it hurts. Just get it over with."

"Open your eyes," Alex replied.

"I can't until you're done," I groaned.

"Betsy, just open them up." Grimacing, I turned my head, opened one eye, and much to my surprise, the empty syringe was in front of my face. "I'm done. It's over," he smiled. My eyes wide with wonder, I threw my arms around his neck and we laughed and laughed. Alex was pretty proud of himself, and I was proud of him. Maybe he should rethink medical school, I teased.

On Monday, I was to have the angiogram, a procedure which detects blockages by moving a catheter through the blood vessels. Normally the catheter is inserted through a small incision in the groin area, but because I had been on blood thinners and had taken Zevalin five days earlier, Dr. Kaminski ordered the catheter to enter through an IV in my arm. Sandy, his nurse, inserted the IV and attached a tube through which the catheter could wind through my body.

On the way to the radiology department, I fully expected that I would get three or four brains for the price of one. What I didn't expect was for entertainment to be thrown in for free. Once I had stretched out on the table in the dimly lit room, two people entered through the rear door. I recognized one as a nurse, but the other wore apparel I had never seen before. The young man's head was covered with an oversized baby blue hat with an elastic band around its perimeter. The hat complimented his baby blue vest and matching knee-length skirt, both fashioned of what I presumed to be trendy hospital fabric—lead. Below the skirt, several inches of hairy legs extended to black socks and shoes. Thinking that this young man's coordinated outfit was at least somewhat more fashionable than the hospital gown I wore, I considered asking him if he would like to swap, but he had already introduced himself and begun to explain the procedure. And then he noticed the tube dangling from the IV in my arm.

"Oh," he exclaimed excitedly. "I've never done this through the arm." Turning to the nurse, he asked, "What size line do we use for this?" She didn't know.

He told me to stay put and that he would be right back. Like I was going somewhere, I thought. Within moments, he returned with another young man who wore an identical outfit, but who knew no more about the line size than he did. Both were very excited about learning a new way to perform the procedure, though. Again, the first young man told me to stay put and that he would return shortly, and again he returned with another young man who wore the same ensemble. By now, the three blue-skirted, hairy-legged triplets huddled together, studying the tube affixed to my arm with great fascination, and it was all I could do to refrain from bursting out laughing. I knew very well that these young men were residents and that their attending physician would soon join us, but I offered to help anyway. "Hey, if you guys can round up a manual, I'll read it to you while you work."

All three lifted their heads and stared at me as blankly as Alex does when I wisecrack—which amused me even more. And then one of them said, "We don't have a manual. We have Dr. Cho." That was it for me. My laughter was uncontainable, especially since Dr. Cho arrived at that very moment wearing a blue vest and a skirt that hung to his ankles. I almost asked if radiology residents get long skirts instead of diplomas for graduation, but I kept that one to myself.

The hardest part of the whole procedure was trying to stay still when I wanted to shake with laughter—which, of course, is not the best thing to do when a catheter is winding through your heart. When it was all over, the Blue Skirts had found nothing unusual, and the blood thinners were history.

Alex pretended to pout when I told him he'd have to close his medical practice. No more shots. No more tests. And no definitive reason for the pain. Using its astonishing array of tools, medical science had determined, through the process of elimination, that I had no bone cancer, no blood clots, and no interior disorder other than the one we already knew about. That was great news. As it turned out, the pain would take four weeks to subside on its own, and its cause was never found. Our mysterious bodies sometimes outwit even the best doctors—even the ones who actually try to find causes for symptoms.

One week later, after six weeks on Decadron, I was ordered off the stuff cold turkey. That drug should be renamed Industrial Strength No-Doz. For the previous four weeks, I'd averaged only a couple of hours of sleep a night, and then jittered as if I had consumed about five hundred cups of coffee during the remaining hours. I wasn't sorry to eliminate this legal speed from my daily diet, but no one told me I'd turn into Rip Van Winkle when I did.

Two days after I stopped the medication, I slept for thirty-six hours straight. And for the next five weeks, I slept nine to ten hours each night in addition to napping once or twice a day. Between sleep, overwhelming fatigue thwarted my attempts to resurface into the life I had once known. I didn't dare make the forty-five minute drive, one way, into our Detroit-area suppliers. I didn't dare commit to a meeting that was not absolutely necessary. My expectations of returning to our normal life far exceeded reality. My body required time to heal from the cumulative effect of several months of chemotherapy followed so closely by radioimmunotherapy.

Each week at the new hospital, my blood would surrender the secrets of my internal affairs. The secret part was the problem. During all the months that blood was drawn at U of M, Judy had always let me know its status by phone or by email within a matter of hours, another gesture that said, "We're watching out for you. You have enough to worry about without waiting and worrying about test results." At the other hospital, no one ever called, except the time that Dr. Doom had waited two days to inform me of the rise in my lymphocyte count. No doubt Judy had spoiled me, but I was at least confident that someone was looking at the results of the tests. At the other hospital, I had to wait days and then beg for someone to copy the reports. Not only did I wonder what my blood was doing, but I also wondered if anyone ever looked at the reports. Hence, I always sent them to Judy. At least I knew she'd look out for me. And she did. My counts were behaving properly, but we'd have to wait for a CT scan to know whether Zevalin was working.

During the fourth week after treatment, Alex came home from work and went straight to the sink to wash his hands, just as he does every day. He stopped suddenly, thrust his wet hands into his pockets, pulled them out disbelievingly, and thrust them in again. "What are you doing?" I asked.

His color faded and his words could scarcely form. "I just realized my wedding ring is gone. I had it this morning," he mumbled, staring at his empty ring finger.

I put my arms around him and whispered, "Oh Alex, it's only a ring. We'll either find it or replace it. Don't worry." He did worry. That ring was the tangible, permanent possession that would outlast me.

We searched his truck, and for days, he retraced his steps and searched jobsites with his metal detector, but the ring was gone. It couldn't possibly have fallen from his finger. For months I had watched him fidget with it, twisting it around and around and then pulling it slightly over his knuckle and pushing it back again. Somewhere we suspected he had pulled it over his knuckle once too often. He couldn't have felt much worse.

During the fifth and sixth weeks after Zevalin, I slept less during the day, and I regained some of the energy I had given up to fight the Invisible Invader. My hair began to sprout, and I giggled when I brought my razor out of retirement, changed the blade and shaved my legs for the first time in months. The fog began to lift from chemo brain, and I could remember what day it was and recite paragraphs in our building contract. Alex and I were pleased, and our optimism grew stronger each day.

There was, however, one small dilemma. I'd lost interest in everything about my job. The process of building homes was no longer exciting. Homes themselves became shelters from the elements. Nothing more. Nothing less. Choosing sinks and windows and carpet and tile seemed utterly insignificant. If a tub held water, what more could anyone want? No sense agonizing over the make and model. Intellectually, I knew how exciting building a new home can and should be, and I had always been passionate about helping our clients through every phase, but the Invisible Invader had replaced my passion with apathy. How would I regain my interest? Or would I?

By October 28, when I walked into the hospital for a CT scan, I couldn't help but wonder if all the effort had been worth it. What would the pictures reveal? Dr. Kaminski called to report the news, his voice resounding with pleasure as he related that all lymph nodes were within normal range. I grinned from ear to ear. For now, Zevalin had defeated the Invisible Invader. Six weeks wasn't a long time, much too early to consider using the word "remission," but Dr. Kaminski and I agreed that for now, I was on vacation from cancer. And *that* was good enough for me.

CHAPTER TWELVE

LETTING GO AND GOING ON

At last I realized what Dr. Kaminski's words had really meant during our first meeting all those months ago. Figuratively, he had said, "Cancer is a winding, obstacle-laden road, but we are here to guide you. Here, take our hands. We will firmly hold yours and lead you, as best we can, to recovery." I had taken the many hands that had reached out to me and gratefully held on for dear life.

Now we had arrived at our destination and it was time to let go. But how? Physically, I was on my way to recovering my old energy, but I was now traveling the road alone. My old busy life loomed somewhere in the distance, yet it eluded me as I stumbled toward it. My *self* had to learn to live in the same body that had just tried to kill me. How could I trust it not to pull that same stunt again?

I'd spent endless hours fantasizing about how life would be after treatment ended, and I was ecstatic that it had ended, but just what was I supposed to do now? In the few seconds it had taken Dr. Ketcham to say, "We suspect lymphoma," life as I'd known it had ceased. He'd hardly spoken the words before day-to-day life became a whirlwind of tests, appointments, treatments, and side effects. There was always someone to tell me where to go, what to do, and when to do it. Robotically, I had followed every instruction and concentrated on getting well. Then, in the few seconds it had taken Dr. Kaminski to say, "It's over," the goal on which I had focused for ten months ceased to exist. Just like that. Gone. Poof. Not that I wasn't glad, but what purpose did I have now?

And just where *was* my old self—the self that had once consisted of many pieces scattered far and wide to make me complete? When cancer had called, I had quickly gathered all my pieces to focus on reaching a single goal, a goal which no longer existed. Suddenly, all the things that I had ignored during my illness were back and important again, but how would I disassemble my "single purpose" self and return to the multiple roles I had once played? And just what was I supposed to talk about at a social or business function? The latest cancer article I'd read? Hawkeye's escapades? How excited I was to be able to stay awake all day?

The physical battle was over, but it seemed that the Invisible Invader had won after all. It had usurped my momentum, stolen my passion, and left me in an emotional vacuum from which I knew not how to escape. How ironic, I thought, that miraculous drugs could rid my body of something so invasive as cancer and still leave me feeling so vulnerable. So timid. So empty. I guessed the doctors had no antidote for that. I'd have to find it myself. But where? And how?

Somehow I had to put all this into perspective. I told

myself that I was still the same person—not just a person who had once had cancer. I reminded myself that I was the sum of all my parts and that the Invisible Invader had only been a part of slightly less than one fifty-second of my entire life, a small fraction within that much longer span. And yet, it left more scars and doubts than any experience that preceded it. A previous divorce or cold don't predict a future divorce or cold. Cancer is different. It predicts a future that holds frequent tests and potentially unimaginable medical procedures. How was I to learn to live with uncertainty as my constant companion?

And had cancer really been a "journey," as it is often described? From the beginning, "journey" had never sounded like an accurate description, and I'd often thought, "If cancer is a journey, I want a new travel agent." Cancer was a destination to which I had never wanted to journey in the first place. I preferred to think of *life* as a journey. Cancer was just a bad detour to an awful place that had robbed me of my physical well-being, my freedom, my confidence, my dreams, and my ability to protect the people I love the most from fear and worry. I don't recommend booking a reservation, but somehow I'd have to face the distinct possibility that my body would book another one for me.

Any hint of pain, any twitch sent me into a tizzy of fear. The same girl who had once ignored every little ache and pain now overreacted to each and every one. If I broke a fingernail, lymphoma was surely back. Okay, I wasn't *that* neurotic, but I came close. I still feared that going into crowds could expose me to germs and send me straight back to Hotel Hell. And the absence of weekly blood draws meant that I had no idea if my own blood was scheming against me. If my medical team was no longer watching out for me, who was? As long as I was being treated, people were working hard to save my life, and I was safe from harm. Now what?

And how could I possibly re-establish myself as dependable? I knew how much Alex had shouldered during my illness, and I genuinely wanted to remove the extra load from him, but I couldn't muster any interest in work. Ever so gently, Alex tried to coax me back by including me in meetings and asking my opinion about a variety of things. I participated, but only half-heartedly, and only because I felt badly that Alex had carried my share of the load for so many months. He was incredibly patient. Had I been in his shoes, I might have screamed at me, "Listen, lady, you've been sick. It's over. Get a grip." I repeated those words to myself over and over again, but it didn't help.

By mid-November, I consciously set myself up to take small steps toward normalcy. I forced myself to accomplish something every day at work. I dared to go to lunch with a friend and silently cheered when I only thought—not panicked—about germs lurking in the restaurant's kitchen. Alex and I invited friends for dinner and delighted that cancer was a mere footnote to the conversation.

I ventured back onto our jobsites more regularly and ran into subcontractors I hadn't seen in months. Each and every one told the same story. They were happy to see me alive and well. Alex had looked exhausted and hadn't been himself for months. Sometimes he'd told them to do one thing when something else was needed. As one of them told me, "We just ignored the old boy and did what we knew he meant."

Alex and I put our house back on the market, and I was proud that I could manage to keep it in showing condition every day. I still dreaded dismantling one house and setting up another, but considering everything else we had gone through, moving was a minor inconvenience. We would sell it in five weeks.

On Thanksgiving, we had eleven people for dinner. I thoroughly enjoyed cooking far more food than we could eat and engaging in lively conversation with family and friends. More than any year before, we had so very much for which to be thankful.

By the end of November, a whole month had passed without my calling Judy for a single ailment, even when I ran a slight temperature for a day mid-month. Most days, however, I could scarcely resist the urge to call and ask, "Are you *sure* I'm okay? May I *please* have a blood test just to make sure?" And yes, this is the same person who hated needles just a few months earlier. I still hate them, but those internal audits had kept us all informed about what my blood was doing, and I wondered what shenanigans it might pull if we weren't watching.

Early in December, I was immensely relieved to have blood drawn, another CT scan, and to see Dr. Kaminski and Judy again. In the reception area, I commented to Alex about how our perception of waiting for them had changed during the year. At first exasperated by any appointment that pulled us from our own schedules, we had quickly become quite unperturbed if they were running late, knowing that a schedule gone awry simply meant that they were taking their time to help each individual patient with his or her own special needs, and that they would do the same for me when our turn came. I was quite grateful that assembly line medicine was never practiced at the Lymphoma Clinic.

Dr. Kaminski and Judy gave me a thorough inspection and reported that the pictures looked great. Wow—three months had passed with no sign of the Invisible Invader! Dr. Kaminski and Judy beamed. I beamed with them and thought how nice it was for them to see the fruits of their labor and to deliver good news for a change. I also teased Alex that we should put those CT scan pictures on our Christmas cards.

I asked Dr. Kaminski how long we could expect the Zevalin to last and what options we would have if it stopped working. Of course, there's no way of knowing how long the disease will stay away, but based on experience with his Bexxar patients whose diseases were as chemo-resistant as mine was, Dr. Kaminski told us that we could reasonably hope for a couple of years. He added that the time frame could move farther out, depending on the depth of remission over the next several months. And if the disease returns, we may or may not have other options before proceeding to a bone marrow transplant. I'm still determined to defy the odds and the medians.

Alex and I met with Dr. Voravit Ratanatharathorn of the Blood and Marrow Transplant Unit on December 3. Emotionally, that meeting was both a setback and an awakening. As I had read, the procedure is risky and unpleasant, and it requires a lengthy stay in Hotel Hell and an even more lengthy recovery period at home. And if it fails, I'm a goner. Dr. Ratanatharathorn and Dr. Kaminski decided that we will proceed to the transplant only if necessary, but I'm scared to death that I may someday have to face that option. And just now, I'm not ready for another fight. I'm still licking my wounds from the last one. But just as I promised Alex, the door remains open.

Until our consultation, I hadn't realized that U of M was searching so hard for a donor, but we learned that they had found one. Only one. Out of eight million. Transplant patients aren't allowed to know the identity of their donors until one year has passed after the transplant, but we did learn that my donor is a forty-one-year-old man who lives in another country. Even this small amount of information immediately made that man a very real human being, and I wept with joy when I thought of him. He would be told that my medical condition had improved and his donation wasn't needed at the moment. I prayed that he would be available if it is.

Alex and I went out for dinner after our consultation. At the restaurant, tears were still spilling down my cheeks. I couldn't stop thinking about this man who was willing to donate his marrow so that I might have a chance to live—

a man I have never met and who would receive nothing for his donation. Can any human being be more unselfish? I think of this stranger each and every day, and tears well up when I do. I wish I could send a message to let him know how deeply I am touched by his selfless generosity.

The consultation again raised all the uncertainty I would have to learn how to face. Fear of becoming bedridden crept in. Of becoming dependent. And useless. And of dying. It was time to have another heart-to-heart with myself. I asked myself if my future—or anyone's—comes with a guarantee. No, it doesn't. If I worried about becoming bedridden or undergoing horrible future treatments, would worrying change the outcome? No. Would worrying today about things I couldn't control tomorrow make me miserable? Yes. And if I were miserable, wouldn't everyone around me be miserable too? Yes. Did I want that? No. Could I set goals and work each day to reach them? Yes. Could I focus on each day and do one, maybe two or three, things to make someone else happy? Yes.

And if the cancer were to return? I knew that I wouldn't fight the battle alone, but with the companionship of family and friends, with the best scientific resources available, and with the most compassionate medical team I could ever have imagined. I knew that Dr. Kaminski and Judy would never, ever, leave me dangling or wondering what's next. As grim as it sounded, I could just hear them reassuring me at the end that there was nothing more they could do medically, but that they would do everything possible to make me comfortable. They always did offset bad news with something good, a concept that every health care professional should practice.

Oh, I was being so strong and so reasonable, I told myself. Couldn't I ever allow myself to wallow in a little self-pity? Okay, self, you can have that luxury. Just don't let it last long.

I quickly concluded that fear of future uncertainties could easily rob me of present joys. When fears crept in, I consciously fought to push them aside. I got busy at work. Called a friend. Took a walk. Listened to whatever music made me happy at the time. Baked a cake and gave it away. Called Alex and told him I loved him. Looked at pictures of Skye and Nicholas. I did whatever it took to banish the uncertainties at any given moment, and sometimes the effort was far more difficult than it had been during treatment. But the price of giving up was far too high.

During the second week in December, Alex called from one of our jobsites for clarification about a client's tile selection. Without hesitation, I told him to stay there and that I would meet him in five minutes. On the drive over, I realized that this was the old me! I hadn't just answered Alex's question on the phone. I'd jumped in my car to visually show him what would have been nearly impossible to explain on the phone. Sensing my old interest returning, we both smiled broadly when I arrived.

The following week, Alex and I were studying plans for a spec home we would soon begin. He suggested eliminating a small, second-floor balcony with its balustrades. Wide-eyed, I implored, "Alex, you *have* to build that balcony. Those balustrades *make* the whole front of the house. You *can't* eliminate them."

Grinning from ear to ear, he snickered, "Maybe I liked it better when you were asleep." I was back, caring about every component in our homes.

On December 17, an advisory panel to the FDA at last recommended approval for Bexxar, the first step in final approval. Alex and I heard the news the following morning, and that night, Beethoven's Ninth Symphony, "Ode to Joy," seemed an appropriate accompaniment to the toast we made to Dr. Kaminski's success.

Two days later, we joyously flew to West Palm Beach for the first time in a year. By then I'd nearly completed this manuscript and had wanted to include Alex's feelings as well as mine. Throughout the year, when I had asked how he felt about this or that, he'd almost always responded, "We'll do what we have to do," "Don't worry about me," or some equally unrevealing comment. But how did he *feel?*

Alex had promised that I could interview him in Florida so that I could sprinkle his comments throughout the manuscript after our conversations. We agreed that no question would be off limits—except one. I couldn't ask him if he'd ever cried. "Well, *did* you?" was my natural question.

"If I did, I won't admit it," he replied with a half-cocked smile.

For a man who likes to remain private, strong, and always in control, and one who naturally looks forward and not backward, I had thought that it would be difficult for Alex to reflect on and admit the fear and anxiety that had often overwhelmed him, especially knowing that he would be revealing himself not only to me, but also to family, friends, and strangers. But in a giant leap, he finally broke his stoic, just-the-facts-ma'am silence. He answered every question I asked and many that I didn't, hoping that his revelations would be helpful to someone who may wear his uncomfortable shoes someday. To me, there was no great revelation. I had suspected everything Alex told me and was proud that he articulated his feelings better than I ever suspected he would.

Throughout the next several days, Alex and I strolled the beach and sat by the pool reflecting on the past year. As bad as it had been, we knew that we had been among the luckiest of the unlucky. In the emergency room, what if Dr. Ketcham had turned to the more "important" traumas of the evening and dismissed my fever as something that would resolve on its own? When it did several days later, I would not have gone to another doctor. Still feeling fine by the time I began chemo in April, how much more trouble would I have been in by the time another symptom appeared?

And what if we hadn't lived in Ann Arbor? Of course there would have been other hospitals, but how lucky we were to live so close to one of the best. And we'd learned that a teaching hospital is meteorically different than what we had imagined. Of course the ranking and financial future of any teaching hospital is dependent on its research, but everyone I met at U of M seemed to clearly understand that *people* were their most valuable resource, mice and monkeys notwithstanding. Everyone seemed infinitely conscious that they were, in fact, treating people. Not lymphoma. Not pneumonia. Not broken arms.

No, I was never treated as a statistic or as a contributor to research. No one ever let cancer define me as a human being. Had Dr. Kaminski merely prescribed medications, my body would most likely have healed the same way, but my psyche would have come away far more injured. He and Judy and Carolyn included sensitivity, intuition, and nurturing as an important part of the whole treatment, a part that buffered the falls and lifted me to heights to which I would never have risen without it. By sharing the suffering of another human being, no doubt surrendering their own comfort at times to do so, they helped me to *live*, not simply exist, through the illness, and they taught me that medicine, done right, is profoundly personal. Alex and I agreed that their healing power had transcended the science of medicine.

We also knew, of course, that physicians make difficult, life-and-death decisions and must therefore remain emotionally unattached in order to maintain the level-headedness to do so. Yet we marveled at the balance Dr. Kaminski and his colleagues had struck between remaining detached and caring so profoundly. How he and Judy and all the others faced the horrors of cancer day in and day out was beyond our comprehension. We were deeply grateful that they could.

At last I understood our relationship, and it turned out to be just as I had expected—unlike any other I have ever had. I learned very little personally about the people who worked so hard to save my life, but I came to realize that it didn't matter. They gave me the best of themselves relative to my needs, and that's what matters. We genuinely grew to like Dr. Kaminski and Judy, and in another time and place, perhaps we might have found common interests besides lymphoma, but the professional relationship we forged is far more important than their friendship. After all, we may need their cool, professional heads to prevail someday. And if we do, we're confident that they'll be around if we need them, and confident that others in the clinic will treat us as they do if an emergency arises in their absence.

And no, Alex and I don't always expect them to be around. We wouldn't want them to be on call 24/7, for me or for anyone else. We genuinely believe that if we—their patients—are to expect the best from our doctors and nurses when they are working, then it seems that they, like everyone else, need time away from us to recharge their batteries. I know. I live with a workaholic who is the first to admit that he is far more effective at work after every little infrequent break I can persuade him to take.

And that exclusive little medical boutique we had stumbled into months earlier? At the Lymphoma Clinic, treatment—medical and psychological—was truly custom tailored. The unique qualities of every patient were clearly recognized and respected. No one ever had a canned script. Instead, Dr. Kaminski and Judy had quickly sized up my personality at our first meeting and had tailored subsequent conversations accordingly. Some months into treatment, I finally figured out what they were doing and found it somewhat entertaining that some of the very working-with-people training I'd taken over the years was being used on me, and it made an enormous difference in how I responded to them and to the illness. In my humble opinion, all health care professionals should sneak out of medical school for a good seminar on understanding personality differences and delivering good customer service.

Yes, we had been lucky in so many ways, Alex and I thought. We'd had excellent insurance, no small children to further complicate matters, the flexibility that self-employment allowed, supportive family and friends, and each other. Still, cancer had invaded every aspect of our lives, and it had exacted a huge toll. Financially, our business goals had fallen far short of what we had expected for the year, but the good news was, we still had a business. Emotionally, Alex and I had neither sunk so low as some nor coped as well as others. As best we could, we'd simply muddled our way through a range and depth of emotions we could never have imagined before cancer, and thankfully, our marriage had withstood the pressures.

Alex and I agreed that the difference between past emotions and disease-related ones was a matter of intensity. During my illness, I wasn't just tired—I was exhausted. Annual celebrations—birthdays and anniversaries—were cause for a national holiday. A routine cookout with family and friends turned into a veritable feast. And I joked, "Yeah, the fear of losing my life *was* a tad stronger than the fear of losing a sale."

Strolling the beach one day, I asked Alex if he still

thought about cancer every day. "Yeah, I do," he sadly admitted. "I don't worry so much anymore, but . . . " his voice drifted off.

"But *what?*" I asked.

After a few silent moments, he finally confided, "Okay. I know this isn't over yet. Sure, a truce has been called, and I pray the truce will last a very long time. But I can't completely push the thoughts aside. I wish I could."

I squeezed Alex's hand and confided my same fears. "I wonder if the Invisible Invader will always be lurking in the background. When someone strikes up a conversation with 'How are you?' I wonder if I will ever be able to answer, 'Fine, thanks,' without silently adding, 'Except for the fact that I have a chronic disease called lymphoma and I might get a fever again one day and then I'll have to hightail it back to the doctor and find out if I need a bone marrow trans-plant and then I might die.' " Alex squeezed my hand back.

By the pool one afternoon, I said to Alex, "You know, we've never resolved what will happen if I get sick again. We really do need a backup plan." Alex reminded me that he had only agreed to divulge his feelings about the previous twelve months. I pushed. "So what will happen if I land in the hospital one day?"

"I'll deal with it if I have to," he said firmly.

I pressed harder. "Alex, you buy car insurance. It doesn't mean you'll ever need it, but you wouldn't drive without it. Making a plan is the same thing."

Alex sat up slightly in the lounge chair, looked over the top of his sunglasses, and refused to address the question.

"Look, once we finish Mystic Ridge, I'm gonna slow down and take you to Bequia and teach you how to hoist a sail."

Hadn't Alex just admitted that he still thinks of cancer every day? I realized then that he needed a rest, some time to heal before he faced future complications. Was I being fatalistic—or simply realistic? Knowing that he had no intention of helping to "put our affairs in order" at that moment, I teasingly replied, "You? Slow down? I *gotta* live to see this."

We changed the subject and talked about how our hopes had changed. Sitting by the same pool a year earlier, we'd made plans for our upcoming developments and hoped for their success. How quickly those grand, self-serving, long-term goals had been dwarfed by smaller, short-term ones. We'd first hoped that the doctors were wrong, and when they weren't, that CVP would succeed. Then that CHOP would succeed. That side effects would be minimal. That each blood test and CT scan would yield good results. That a bad day would turn into a good tomorrow. Little hopes, one after another, had saved us from emotional bankruptcy.

Sitting by the same pool a year later, we hoped only that my body would remain healthy and strong. Everything else paled in comparison. But then Alex teased, "Okay, you've had your year off. The roads are going in at Mystic Ridge and you've got 177 houses to sell. Can we pick up where we left off a year ago?"

I groaned and teased back, "Does that mean I really have to go back to work? I kinda liked semi-retirement." Then I added jokingly, "You know, we don't have to wait until we finish Mystic Ridge. We could go to Bequia in February. And Paris is nice in the spring. And how about St. Petersburg in the summer? And—"

"Betsy, did you just win the lottery? Or just how many houses can you sell by February?"

With a melodramatic sigh and a toss of my head against the lounge chair, I moaned, "Oh, I can't sell any. I'm just too tired. Wake me up when it's time to pack."

"Well, I guess we can't go anywhere since you're so tired." Why did I always back myself into corners?

During a lull in one of our many conversations, I lay back to absorb the sun's warmth and thought about how Alex had coped. We had debated about who had suffered more, and he believed that I did. I disagreed. I'd had a brief preview of the medical world. He'd had none. I had taken more drugs than a couple of hippies and they'd kept me asleep much of the time, or at least detached from my responsibilities, all of which he'd carried. I'd received treatment and attention while he'd watched helplessly from the sidelines.

And cancer had definitely complicated his life. He'd had a business to run and employees who depended on our success to feed their families. He'd had his children Greta and Zan to think about. He couldn't possibly have let himself go down. At the same time, cancer had also forced him into the demanding role of supporting someone who has a major illness, a role no one is ever prepared to play. And yet when I was diagnosed, he responded with every ounce of his energy, better than most people could have. He stopped his life many times in order to help me rescue mine. While everyone else saw my brave and funny face, he bore the brunt of my emotions from their highest highs to their deepest lows, and always, he was my wall against the crush of them.

How he had maintained his composure day after day seemed remarkable. I was amazed that he had found that delicate balance between fighting the battle with me and not being consumed by it. If the roles had been reversed, I seriously doubt I could have managed as well as he did. My emotional survival and ultimate recovery is as much his victory as it is mine.

But where does all this leave us? It leaves us hoping that scientists will continue working around the clock to find cures for me and for every other family whose life is derailed by disease. It leaves us hoping that Zevalin will work long enough for another therapy to become available should I need it. It leaves us hoping that we will have many good years together even as we make each day the best that it can be.

And it leaves me living in two time zones simultaneously. I reside in real time where I have responsibilities and I care about all things big and small, from work to washing the floors. In real time, I sometimes get irritated that the demands of the moment grab my attention, change my schedule, and expect me to make instant decisions and responses when I would prefer to savor the moment, to slow life down a bit. But I also live in lymphoma time where a sense of urgency cries out, "Someday is now. Hurry up."

In real time, I wish I'd had dry rot. Or chiggers. Or a yeast infection. I wish God would ban cancer and every other disease. But the lymphoma zone leaves little time to wish for that which I cannot change or even to spend much energy worrying about the outcome of my illness. The outcome of my *life* seems far more significant.

On Christmas Day, I handed Alex a small gift which he slowly unwrapped. Inside was the ring box that had once held his ring. It was empty except for a note that read, "Dear Alex, Tomorrow we will go size your new ring. I love you, Betsy." His bottom and top lips curled toward the inside of his mouth, and he stared silently at the note for several long moments. Pulling me close, he finally stammered, almost inaudibly, "I'm sorry I lost . . . I wish . . . You shouldn't . . . " Silence again.

"You're welcome. Glad you like it," I spoke for him.

And then he asked, "Could we have the ring inscribed just like the old one?"

The following day, we headed to Michael's Jewelers in downtown West Palm Beach where my friends Michael and Murray Sperber were expecting us. I gave them all the necessary artwork to emblazon the coat-of-arms on the ring, and Alex wrote the inscription for engraving on the inside: *ESH to ATdeP, 9-6-98*. Michael jokingly offered to insert a pin through Alex's finger *and* the ring. Half smiling, Alex turned to me and said, "*You* just need to stay well so I don't fidget."

I saluted him. "Yes, dear." Neither of us had to say that I had just put one of my affairs in order. And so, I added lightly, "Lose it again and *your* life will be in danger."

On December 30, we were to return to Ann Arbor on a very early morning flight. Packing up the night before, I encouraged Alex to do likewise but he was too busy reading a book. I pressed, "Alex, why don't you take a break and pack up tonight so we won't be rushed in the morning?"

"Don't worry," he mumbled, paying no attention to me.

Absentmindedly, I said, "Alex, you're gonna be late for your own funeral."

He started to answer, "Yeah, but . . . " then stopped, put the book down, and looked horrified.

Before he could say anything, I laughed and finished the sentence for him. "Yeah, I know, I'm gonna be early to mine."

"Betsy, I'm sorry, I didn't mean to . . . No, you can't be early. I mean . . . "

"Alex, it's just an expression. We've said it for years. You're always late. I'm always early—or at least on time. What's gonna change?"

Grimacing, he suggested, "How about a new expression?"

"Be on time and we won't need one," I bantered with a smile.

Waiting to board the plane the following morning, I was reading *Sunlight At Midnight*, a book about the history of St. Petersburg which Alex had given to me for Christmas. Without warning, my eyes flooded with tears and my chin began to quiver. Russian history may have its tragic moments, but it's not *that* tragic, I thought. What was wrong with me? There was that little voice again asking whether or not I would be able to return to Florida for another Christmas. It told me I'd never get to St. Petersburg. This time, I shot back. "Don't bet on it. I have lots of frequent flier miles left."

Trying to stop the tears, I looked up at the ceiling and hated my subconscious for interrupting a perfectly good book, for reminding me of nagging doubts, *and* for doing it in a public place. I turned to Alex, who saw my moist eyes and thought I was sad about leaving Juli and the babies, and I began a conversation about work. I knew I could talk louder and faster than those doubts, and I did. They were soon gone.

Back in Ann Arbor, we stayed awake to watch the ball drop on New Year's Eve. As 2003 rang in, we held each other close and Alex whispered, "A new year. A fresh start. Thank God." And I *did* thank God.

On January 7, I awakened at five-thirty to a full schedule. I poured myself a cup of coffee. Alex and I discussed the day's plans. I checked email and cursed, then deleted, eighty-three spams. I answered messages from Noreen and a client. Got dressed and put the wig on, then took it off. Screw it, I thought. I'm tired of the damn thing. I looked in my vanity for mousse, spiked my *very* short hair, and left the house, wigless, for the first time in months. I drove up US-23 toward our tile supplier while wishing I were on my way to have a blood test instead. I turned the music up louder and let Ukrainian folk music nudge my thoughts from the hospital and carry me to Lviv. I passed the Silver Lake exit and thought about Dr. Ketcham's call exactly one year earlier. I smiled as I remembered his response when I'd recently run into him and thanked him for being so thorough. He'd modestly said, "No thanks necessary. I was just doing my job."

In the afternoon, I met a client and our kitchen designer. Snow covered the ground. Even in the new coat I had just bought—on sale—I nearly froze as we laid out the kitchen in the open frame of the house. Afterward, as I drove to meet another client, Jimmy Buffett's tropical music was just what I needed to warm me. I slipped in a CD and idly began humming along, preoccupied with thoughts of my next meeting. Suddenly, Jimmy himself may as well have been sitting in the passenger seat saying, "Hey, listen up. This one's for you, babe." Loud and clear, he sang out, "Yesterday's over my shoulder, so I can't look back for too long. There's just so much to see waiting in front of me that I know that I just can't go wrong . . . With these changes in latitude, changes in attitude, nothin' remains quite the same. For all of our runnin' and all of our cunnin'—if we couldn't laugh, we would all go insane."

Y-e-e-e-s-s-s! *There's just so much to see waiting in front of me!* I replayed that part of the song over and over again, all the way to my next meeting. And every time Jimmy sang, "There's just so much to see waiting in front of me," I bellowed out the words with him. Neither chemo nor RIT had improved my vocal skills, but life was good again!

Later that day, I reviewed plans for a Mystic Ridge house, ordered title work for an impending sale, resisted a strong urge to call Judy and *beg* her to order a blood test. I stopped by the grocery store, filled my car with gas, called Alex three, maybe four times to say, "I love you," cooked dinner, lay on the couch watching the news with Tooties purring in my ear, sewed a button on a shirt, and packed a few boxes for our move, just three weeks away. It was a routine day in our life—our *normal* life!

While I was packing boxes in the dining room, Alex wandered in and asked, "You really want to go to St. Petersburg, don't you?"

Without looking up, I answered, "Sure, I'd love to visit the Hermitage and a thousand other places on this earth. Why?"

"Well, let's plan it. How about sometime in July?"

Astonished, I looked up and asked, "Do you mean it? You'd take off work during the busiest time of year?"

Grinning from ear to ear, Alex replied, "Why not?"

I could scarcely believe Alex's words. I can hardly persuade him to take an hour off from work, much less enough time to travel overseas. For a few moments, I was thrilled, until uncertainty tried to steal my delight. "Alex, that's months from now. What if— "

"Betsy, don't you recognize that you're already planning ahead for things? Dr. Kaminski handed our life back to us. We need to let go of the past year and go on."

"Yes, we do," I smiled. "Okay, let's do it. So—if we go to St. Petersburg, we might as well fly down to Lviv and visit your cousin. And if we're that close to Prague—"

"Betsy, plan for a week," Alex chuckled. "Not a month."

"Well, I thought I'd try," I laughed.

When Alex and I crawled into bed that night, we read for a few minutes as we do every night. Had he known what day it was? If he had, he hadn't mentioned it, and I decided not to remind him. He kissed me goodnight, turned out the lights, and fell asleep quickly. The roller coaster we'd ridden for nearly a year had finally ground to a halt and we were back on the ground.

In the darkness, I wondered if I'd make it to Skye's and Nicholas's college graduations and then mused that they'd hardly notice my presence, busy as they would be with their own friends. But just now, they're still young enough to play with their old—make that young—grandmother. Pulling the future a little closer and imagining their smiles and giggles, I dreamt of taking them to Disney World soon. There, the roller coaster is *fun!*

THE HONORABLE DISCHARGE

June 2004. "You leave that hair alone. It's the Blond Badge of Courage," I joked to Alex recently when he absent-mindedly plucked a hair from the shoulder of my black sweater.

"Looks more like your honorable discharge to me," he smiled.

Yep, I have plenty of hair these days. It's a marvelous accessory to good health!

Alex is better, too. His droopy shoulders have straightened. His eyes light up. He smiles his genteel smile much more easily. No permanent lines remain from months of furrowing his eyebrows. He doesn't fidget with his wedding ring. I can't say that cancer made him stop to smell the roses, but he occasionally sniffs a petal or two. Mostly, he's back in full workaholic swing, and these days, he sometimes forgets that the company will survive should we step out on an occasional weeknight. Of course I consider it my wifely duty to remind him, and he smiles sheepishly when I do.

As for me, I feel grand! By spring of last year, my energy

level was about equivalent to what it was when I was diagnosed. By summer, I was peppier than I had been in several years. By fall, people who hadn't seen me in some time commented that I looked better than ever. In retrospect, cancer had been eating away at me for a long time, so slowly and subtly that no one noticed, not even me. But my physical recovery outpaced my emotional one.

When I wrote the last chapter eighteen months ago, I sounded pretty convincing that I was letting go of cancer and going on, didn't I? The truth is, learning to let go of cancer is no different than acquiring any other new skill. It takes time. It takes effort. And it takes repetition until you get it right. We've been practicing all these months, and our skills are improving.

For several months after treatment ended, I consciously, furiously, fought off the gremlins of doubt that cancer had left behind—gremlins that would land on my shoulder and whisper in my ear, "Ha, ha, you may be well now, but every healthy day puts you one day closer to starring in *The Return of the Invisible Invader.*" I spent much time and effort fighting off the gremlins and gradually succeeded in chasing most of them away most of the time. Only occasionally does one appear these days, and I set it straight very quickly. "Yes, I *am* well now," I reply, "and every day puts me one day farther *away* from the Invisible Invader. I have no intention of starring in the sequel."

As much as I fought to jump right back into my old life, I didn't. Hard as I looked, I couldn't find it. Several months would pass before I would realize that my old life, as I once knew it, was long gone. Of course it was. You can't retrieve what is in the past and you can't move forward while you're looking backward. As I gradually began to look ahead, I glimpsed large remnants of my old life rearranged and emerging into a new life. You see, cancer sends you on a slightly different path. It strips away everything but what is most important and leaves you learning how to let go of what is unimportant and how to hold on to what is. Pushed and pulled by the demands of daily life, that isn't always easy, but we've made huge strides.

One step at a time, I returned to most of my old activities, at least the ones to which I wanted to return. And I found some new interests. I learned to make commitments a week ahead, then two, then three. Four weeks out was harder, but I forced myself to make them so long as they kept me close to home. I was perfectly happy to travel in the states, and I did. I visited the grandbabies. Went to a family reunion. Flew down to Florida for Noreen's college graduation. Adulthood had interrupted her earlier educational plans, but she'd returned to school to complete her degree shortly before my stay in Hotel Hell. Lying in the hospital bed, I'd teasingly asked her if she was going to wear cap and gown with all the youngsters. She'd told me, "I'll walk that walk if you promise to get out of here and be there." One year after Hotel Hell, I proudly watched her graduate summa cum laude.

The thought of traveling overseas, however, was daunting. I made all kinds of excuses to postpone making arrangements for our St. Petersburg trip. The simple truth is that July, in January, seemed a lifetime away. In February and March, it didn't seem any closer. And what if I relapsed in Russia? The only Russian words I knew meant hello, goodbye, and son of a bitch. How I learned the latter is a funny story for another day, but it wouldn't be exactly useful if I had to communicate with a Russian doctor.

CT scans, blood work, and physical inspections at three-month intervals confirmed that I was achieving deep remission and that I could reasonably expect radioimmunotherapy to continue doing its job for longer than two years. Even with that good news, based on scientific evidence, I was still occasionally haunted by the six and ten month execution dates that Dr. Doom had set for me. Intellectually, I knew better than to let mere words plague me, but they sometimes did, no matter how hard I fought back, and it never ceased to amaze me that reason and logic could shift so easily to doubt. March 11, six months after Zevalin, came and went quite uneventfully, and I breathed a slight sigh of relief, but still I kept myself tethered close enough to Ann Arbor where I could get help quickly if I needed it.

On the first warm spring day, I ventured into the garden for the first time in nearly two years, and the dirtier I got, the happier I was. When Alex pulled into the driveway late in the afternoon, he stopped his truck near where I was working and leaned out the window. Looking up at him, I shivered at the sight of the unadulterated, unabashed smile spread across his face. I remembered that smile. It was the one he reserved for something that particularly pleased him. Realizing how long it had been since I had seen it, my eyes grew a little watery. Alex leaped out of his truck and walked briskly over to scoop me up in his arms. "Boy, is it good to see you out here," he said.

"Ah, yes," I flirted, pulling away and patting his cheeks with clay-stained hands. "Your very dirty, very healthy girl-friend has spent a delightful day playing in the spores." I was indeed overjoyed to reclaim a pastime that I had once loved, but cancer even left an indelible mark on my gardening habits. Still surrounding myself with plants that live indefinitely, annuals are history, and I doubt I will ever plant another. In their stead, perennials blossom, as if their annual resurrection can pull me toward each new spring. Yes, I admit to adding a few quirky superstitions to my repertoire.

By early May, I cautiously investigated airline tickets and accommodations in St. Petersburg. The city was celebrating its three hundredth anniversary that summer, and hotels had been booked for months. What remained was sky high, and airline tickets had doubled since I had first checked in January. Our trip to St. Petersburg was out. My disappointment was offset by relief—there were still two months left before the second execution date.

In June, the FDA finally approved Bexxar, thirteen years after the first clinical trials. Hooray! I have no idea whether Dr. Kaminski took time out to celebrate his own achievement, but one thing I do know. He's not about to rest on his laurels. He continues to study Bexxar to learn why it works well for most people and why others respond less favorably. Should it be used as a front line therapy or after chemo and/or Rituxan fail? I'll bet he will find the answers to those questions. I know he'll never stop trying.

That same month, Alex and I began to consider an alternate overseas trip for September. We searched the web and found reasonable airline tickets and hotel accommodations. Would I buy them? Nope. Not until I woke up breathing after ten months.

Four days before that anniversary, another CT scan proved that I was just fine. I finally asked Dr. Kaminski if it was safe for us to travel overseas. He thought it was a splendid idea and assured me that I did not need to pack a suitcase full of drugs "just in case."

On July 11, 2003, ten months after Zevalin, Alex and I bought our plane tickets, and I was finally free. Free to plan ahead—months ahead. Free at last to *really* let go and go on, and I mostly did. Yes, I know it seems ridiculous that a few words took such a hold of me, and I'm a little ashamed that I was unable to cast them off as the bunk that they were, but cancer wounds are deep, and words, even when you do your best to cast them aside, can keep those deep wounds festering.

Also in July, a year after my last chemo treatment, I was sitting at a stoplight and turned my head quickly to read a sign. Did I feel my hair move? Cautiously, I shook my head from side to side. Y-e-e-e-s-s-s!!! It moved! Barely. But I *did* feel soft wisps brushing the back of my neck! The light turned green, and I sped off, wildly shimmying my head back and forth, laughing and singing, "There's just so much to see waiting in front of me . . . " I really didn't care if neighboring drivers thought I was crazy. In fact, I wanted to shout out the window, "Hallelujah! My hair moves! I'm *normal!*"

Late in the summer, we learned about a program called the Family Centered Experience which, to my knowledge, is the first of its kind in the nation. It pairs U of M's first year medical students with families who have dealt with all kinds of major illnesses. For two years, the students follow a specific outline, which includes learning how our conditions affect our emotions, our daily routines and our plans for the future. They learn about our hopes and fears and how our cultural beliefs influence our conditions. They ask family members how our illnesses impacted them. They want to know how friends responded. And, they ask, what did your medical team do right and what did they do wrong—and why?

Do you see the future of health care actually including *care* as the important part of treatment that it is? Three cheers to U of M for starting this program! I hope it spreads like wildfire to other medical schools.

Dr. Kaminski and I met on September 22, one year and eleven days past Zevalin. I'd reached a huge milestone, he happily reported. A clear CT scan and perfect bloodwork confirmed *complete* remission. And having achieved that blissful state for a whole year, statistics indicated that I could now reasonably expect a five-year reprieve—or longer—provided Zevalin does what Bexxar is known to do. Better yet, if the Invisible Invader attacks again, I'm not necessarily facing more chemo or a bone marrow transplant. Depending on how it returns, *if* it does, I can take Bexxar—

quick, painless, easy. Talk about a relief! That news pushed those gremlins to the moon! In just a year, what break-throughs scientists had made! And how lucky I thought I was to have had cancer when new treatments are enabling more and more of us to live longer, fuller, and healthier lives. Dr. Kaminski, Judy, and I hugged as we said goodbye that day. They were clearly as pleased with my progress as I was.

The following day, Alex and I left work and responsi-bilities behind for twelve glorious days. We flew to Warsaw where we would spend a single night on our way to Lviv, from whence we would head to Krakow, Prague, and points in between. That first night away, under a clear, star-studded Warsaw sky, we strolled the Old Town Square hand in hand. For a while, we walked in silence. Suddenly, Alex pulled me very close and whispered, "This time last year, did you think we'd ever have a trip like this?"

My eyes filled with tears, and I could barely whisper back, "No." There in the square, surrounded by natives and tourists and lively accordions, two crazy-with-joy Americans stood holding each other, thanking God and Dr. Kaminski and Judy and all of our friends and family—and remark-able drugs. At that moment, I think we finally exhaled after taking deep breaths and holding them for a very long time. Cancer was over, and we emerged as two giddy kids with renewed confidence that our happily-ever-after life could at last resume.

As the immediate terror of cancer diminished, day-to-day life really did return to normal in almost every way. I gradually began to answer "Fine" to "How are you?" without wondering if I really was or if the person asking was probing about my health. Once in a while now, someone raises an eyebrow and asks, "No, *really*, how *are* you?" and I realize that he or she wants to know if I still have cancer. Most of the time, I grin and make some wisecrack like, "If you're wondering if I'm planning to do lymphoma again, no. Let's do lunch instead."

Little by little, I settled comfortably into my old job, not because I felt guilty about the workload on Alex, but because I genuinely enjoy helping people plan their new homes. *And* because I am extraordinarily glad that I can. With Mystic Ridge in full swing now, I am in fact working far more than I was pre-cancer. Most of my friends can't understand why. They tell me they'd be off gallivanting if they'd gone through what I did. I admit to having had occasional delusions of chucking it all and living on a boat in the Caribbean, but my checkbook would have undoubtedly screamed, "You're hallucinating!" Even if it hadn't, I wouldn't really have skipped out, at least not for longer than a couple of weeks. How could I possibly have passed up the opportunity to reclaim one of the largest fragments of my old life, especially when I so desperately needed to replace fear and doubt with purpose and passion?

Yes, Alex and I are once again up to our eyeballs in work. The line between our personal and professional lives will always be hopelessly blurred, but our relationship succeeds because we are both equally committed to it, because we both enjoy what we do more than we dislike its inherent challenges, and because we find interludes for fun. And more than ever before, we realize how much each of us completes the other.

One of our old habits never did resurface. The newscasters, who had once joined us from the time we got home until the time we went to bed, tell their grim tales to other people now. Most of their stories are too tragic for me to hear over and over again. Graphic displays and descriptions of current world violence sicken my stomach. Literally.

My mother continues to be a source of inspiration. This past Christmas day, I took a very early flight to Virginia, arriving by the time she was getting up. Karen and I hadn't told her I was coming, and was she ever surprised! As I left to return home, Mother said, "I hope you didn't come to visit me because you thought this was going to be my last Christmas. I'll be around next year, and I'm going to expect you back." I laughed and thought, "Not only did you give me your longevity genes, you taught me the power of hope." She'll be ninety-five in a couple of months, living proof that no one can predict the length of life.

This past spring, "our" medical students asked us a series of questions about our experiences with doctors. We also discussed how losses in our lives had affected us. Alex's candid remarks took me by complete surprise. I had known that a friend of his had died very quickly from bone cancer when they were both in their mid-twenties. Brain cancer had quickly claimed another friend when they were in their early thirties. Some years ago, Alex had briefly told me about them, but their deaths were way before my time, he'd never dwelled on them, and frankly, I'd never given much thought to them after he'd told me.

Shame on me for forgetting those episodes. That night, he began to talk about Sam and Sandy, and his sadness was obvious to all. At that moment, I finally realized how deeply those previous experiences had affected him. After the students left, he at last told me how scared he really was during my illness. "The only two close friends I ever knew who had cancer both died," he said. "Two for two. And when that nurse mentioned bone cancer, I flashed back to Sandy. He was gone in no time." For the first time in his life, I think, Alex finally talked about the deaths of his friends, friends who were closer to him than I had ever realized. I wish I had known.

I wondered why he hadn't shared more details with me sooner. "It just hurt too much," he said. "I kept telling myself that treatments were better than they were all those years ago, and that somehow you wouldn't be number three." Nearly two years after worrying that Alex would not know how to cope with illness, I learned how deeply his earlier experiences had troubled him during mine. What a burden he had carried alone for so long.

With time and distance from the roller coaster of cancer, we are, more than ever, indebted to the friends and family whose love and support helped us through the emotional upheavals and the daily regimens. We'll always be grateful to Dr. Kaminski and Judy and their colleagues. The medications they prescribed healed my body, and their care, wisdom, and compassion safeguarded my soul and my spirit.

It was a perfect combination that undoubtedly left us as unscarred emotionally as any cancer experience possibly could.

And what still astounds me is the science I learned. Don't get me wrong. I wouldn't know a cell if I saw one. And I didn't grow a left brain, despite all the drugs I took. But cancer at least made me sit up and take notice of science, even if it's with a right-brained perspective. I'm still amazed that it took nearly a century to perfect the theory of radioimmunotherapy before it could be used in mainstream medicine. Can you imagine the number of scientists who had worked on that theory all those years? You gotta love every one of them for dreaming big, daring to fail, and persistently, tirelessly spending their lives searching for and finding small pieces of that very complex puzzle.

Since I've lived in Ann Arbor, I've met a few scientists other than Dr. Kaminski, and I was always struck by the passion each one seemed to feel for his or her work. I remember one in particular who sat across from us at a dinner a couple of years before my illness. On and on she chatted about how she had sliced up livers. For four years. And the more she talked, the more animated she got! Yep, it sorta suppressed my appetite for the perfectly good prime rib on my plate. By the end of dinner, she finally got around to telling us that her group had discovered that whatever they were looking for—it escapes me now—couldn't be found in the direction they were looking. "Isn't it fantastic that it only took four years for us to reach a dead end?" she asked. At the time, I had no way of appreciating that four years of persistence, followed by failure, could indeed send her on a path that would lead to a new discovery.

Last fall, I briefly met another researcher quite by chance. Delivering some documents to one of our clients in a section of the hospital's 107 acres that I hadn't seen before, I walked down one drab corridor and then another, passing lab after windowless lab. Most of the doors were wide open, and I saw men and women of all ages, shapes, sizes, and colors hunched over computers and other odd, expensive-looking equipment. I really did get a little lost, so I poked my head into an open door, apologized for interrupting, and asked for directions. A petite woman looked up, smiled, and in a heavy foreign accent, offered to walk me to my destination. Along the way, I couldn't help but ask what she was doing. She grinned broadly and told me she studied DNA and something else that I didn't understand. Her eyes lit up, and she beamed when she added, "It's for breast cancer. We got to make dat bat disease history." I almost hugged her!

Within those walls, and others like them around the world, she and her colleagues sit in labs day after day, month after month, year after year. They're slicing up livers. Or whatever else they carve up. They're studying DNA and proteins and genes. And monkeys. And mice. And real live human beings who brave new, experimental treatments. All contribute to new discoveries which lead to new therapies which improve the length and quality of life for every man, woman, and child who battles disease. New drugs like Bexxar and Zevalin—and many others—are indeed ushering in a whole new era in cancer treatment, giving many of us a real chance to dance at our grandchildrens' weddings. Is it any wonder that I found those drab halls to radiate with hope?

Today, when I drive past the hospital, I still see it for what it is—a major research facility. But now enlightened, I know that the answers found within its walls benefit patients and families far beyond the city limits of Ann Arbor, and it is indeed a privilege to have met some of the people who have dedicated their lives to giving people like you and me the precious gift of time. Yes, the Dr. Kaminskis of this world became my heroes.

And inspired by my new heroes, I couldn't help but wish that every other cancer patient could share the joy that a second chance bestows, but there didn't seem to be much I could do to contribute to the research that yields that joy. Research, after all, requires disciplined scientific energy and training, of which I had neither. But it also requires money. Lots of money. We didn't have much of that to spare, but we did know about OPM. Other people's money.

An idea began to brew, and this past January, without having a clue how to pull it off, Alex and I decided to launch an annual fundraiser which would benefit the Leukemia/Lymphoma/Bone Marrow Transplant Program at the University of Michigan. We knew we couldn't possibly accomplish such an undertaking alone, and within days, ten others had embraced the idea and volunteered to help. Four of us were cancer survivors. One was a bone marrow donor. The others pitched in because they wanted to, and their participation was all the more meaningful. All of us had worked on various fundraisers, but none of us had experience in establishing one. Nonetheless, the twelve of us envisioned a party on the day of the Kentucky Derby which we would call the Derby Challenge. We would broadcast the race, have an auction, and invite our friends to pay admission. It sounded simple enough.

There was one big problem. We had no way to collect tax-deductible donations. In no time, our local Home Builders Association stepped in with their foundation as the vehicle to collect tax-deductible contributions. The organization's staff tracked the funds and dealt with all the state regulations regarding charitable contributions. That was huge support. With that problem solved, donations of goods, services, and money trickled in. People offered advice and encouragement. Local restaurants agreed to donate the food. Our website designers built and donated a website. A local band would play for beer. Bit by bit, thanks to the dedicated committee members and a generous community, we got everything we needed—except enough RSVPs to ensure success. Two weeks before the party, I was more than slightly panicked.

May 1 dawned cold and rainy. The party was to be held that afternoon under a tent in our yard. By the time it started at four o'clock, buckets of rain were falling, and the temperature was dropping steadily. I wondered if anyone would show up. Two hundred people turned out, and when everything was totaled, over three hundred people had donated $30,760 plus goods and services. If that doesn't prove the goodness of humanity and that collective efforts can make a difference, what does? My head is still spinning from so much generosity and support. Proceeds from the first Derby Challenge will be added to other funds for continuing immunotherapy research—research that somewhere, someday, will give someone the joy of a second chance.

I had no intention of writing about the Derby Challenge for fear of it sounding that we had turned our experience into self-serving publicity. Reluctantly, it is included only because friends who knew about this manuscript repeatedly told me I "must" because it might encourage someone to help their own favorite cause. Clearly, friends prevailed, and though I'm not suggesting that everyone should do what we did, I do hope that the account will demonstrate that ordinary people can often accomplish far more than they think when only they try.

I also believe that anyone who has ever dealt with cancer in any capacity understands that cancer connects you with other people in a way that nothing else can. Cancer graduates are enormously sympathetic to those who unwillingly join our diverse community, and I believe that most of us would do anything we could to reach out to our fellow human beings who face the same agonies that we have faced. We simply reach out in the different ways that present themselves to us, whether it's donating money or making a meal for a friend or simply hugging a caregiver. However insignificant or small any gesture might seem, whatever we do matters to someone. And it all adds up to making a difference. Really.

I recently waltzed into the hospital for another CT scan, confident that all my innards were in perfect working order. Judy, still caring as much as ever, left a message for me the following day confirming what I already knew. My innards were picture perfect! I played the message three times, dancing with joy around the answering machine. Still dancing, I called Alex and played it for him. I really don't worry about relapse anymore. Maybe it's because I'm too busy to think much about it. Maybe it's because the doses of reassurance at regular intervals give me a safety net. Maybe it's because I've learned enough about RIT to know that it can and does work for a very long time. Or maybe it's because I truly believe that I am cured. But hearing good news makes me want to sing and dance and celebrate—so I do! And Alex joins me in his own quiet way, relieved and happy that life is good again.

But am I really cured? Or am I in complete remission? It's a matter of semantics. I prefer the word "cured," but that's not a word scientists use easily. By legal and scientific necessity, they must gather many years of data before they even whisper it. But I've got news for them. Some of Dr. Kaminski's early Bexxar patients are still disease-free after ten, eleven, and even twelve years. With all due respect, I think "cured" is perfectly suitable in those cases, and I intend to remain "cured" for however long it takes for scientists to agree with me—and years beyond that!

But not everyone is so optimistic. In a recent discussion group, a couple of ladies who also had lymphoma looked at me in disbelief when I used the word. "You know it's coming back," said one lady. "It's just a matter of time," said the other. Together they chimed that I was burying my head in the sand.

I emphatically disagree. Neither Dr. Kaminski nor those ladies nor I know with any certainty that the Invisible Invader will strike again. We all know that it could. But isn't it also possible that I could get struck by lightning? Or hit by a truck? Or have a heart attack? Or live to be a hundred? There are endless possibilities about how and when my life will end. But before it does, I have better things to think about. The truth is, I don't know what my next scans will show, but I do know that there is no evidence of disease in my body at the moment. That means I am disease-free. Cured. Just for today. And hopefully many tomorrows. As much as I would love to live indefinitely, I have instead learned to live in peaceful coexistence with the uncertainty of life itself. If that means my head is buried in the sand, then so be it.

Today, Alex and I are still the same people we were before cancer invaded our lives. Only now, cancer is part of who we are, and we look at life through a different lens. Yes, cancer changed our view of the world. Staring at death gave us a heightened appreciation for life. It challenged us to live fully the life that we have and forced us to pay attention to the present moment, which is all we really have and all that really matters. And our new perspective gives us more contentment, more joy, more compassion, more empathy.

Many people have asked if I believe that my outlook

contributed to healing. A year ago, I might have answered a confident yes. Today, I'm not so sure. Why did we lose a friend who was as positive as anyone we've ever met? Why is another not responding to treatment? I think now that I was just lucky enough for a powerful new drug to heal my body. Perhaps my will to live made it more receptive, but who can know for sure? The only thing I can say with any certainty is that my attitude helped me to survive the onslaught of uncertainty.

Alex and I never found a one-size-fits-all formula for surviving cancer emotionally. What worked for us might not work for you, and vice versa. We did, however, learn a few strategies that can help us all ride that roller coaster. Like the choices we make. About what we eat, what we watch, what we read, how we exercise. Yes, choices definitely influence how we respond to cancer, and making conscious choices about what we can control helps to remind us that we have not completely lost control of our lives.

We also learned that medical teams directly affect not only physical health, but emotional survival as well. It is absolutely crucial to have complete trust in your medical team, and yes, we know how difficult it is to turn your life over to total strangers. The task is made easier by setting realistic expectations, both for your doctor and for yourself. It helps to recognize that medicine is as much an art as it is a science. And it especially helps to recognize doctors for what they are—human beings with medical degrees. Like the rest of us, they have unique personalities, and it is imperative to have a comfortable, working relationship with them.

Your life and your well-being are at stake, and you have every right to expect to be treated with dignity and compassion. Cancer presents too many other challenges to settle for anything less.

Alex and I also learned the importance of holding on to our dreams, our hopes, and our faith. As beacons of hope beckoning us toward our own future, they gave us powerful reasons to fight back, and we looked long, hard, and often at those reasons, especially on the days when we would rather have been wallowing in self-pity. Our mantra was, "When you're going through hell, keep going," words Winston Churchill uttered many years ago.

While it is much easier said than done, we tried not to get lost in anticipation of what might come next, and instead to focus on each day as it came. To set short-term, achievable goals and to savor the little successes. Because even the little ones add up to big ones.

And each day, we consciously tried to find something, however small, for which to be thankful. Some days it was hard to find anything, but searching for positives helped to offset the negatives. To name but a few items I included on my "Things I am Thankful For" list, aside from family and friends, there were Hershey kisses, sunshine, sunsets, thunderstorms, peaches, Key lime pie, anti-nausea drugs, old family photographs, life's little conveniences like dishwashers and covered parking when it's snowing, my favorite pair of purple heels, and instant-dry nail polish.

As difficult as it sometimes was, we tried to forget the statistics. Statistics are only numbers, and we kept telling ourselves that numbers couldn't kill me. And statistics define large groups of people. They don't define what happens to each individual. And so, instead of dwelling on the statistics of lymphoma, we tried to remember that miracles happen. Indeed, they do.

Finally, we found that panic and fear and despair were perfectly appropriate sometimes. Ask Alex today, and even he will admit to shedding tears on more than one occasion. The key to emotional survival is to panic or cry, and then to face the issue and move on. Laughter helps, and we would encourage you to find whatever it is that makes you laugh. As often as possible. Because it's a wonderful transport to lift you from despair, if only for a moment. Another antidote to sadness is the joy that comes from giving to others, and even during illness, it is still possible to give in words and deeds. More importantly, support groups, counselors, social workers, or clergy lend valuable support, and even the most private people can benefit from sharing the emotional burden of cancer.

Throughout the past several months, many people have told us, "We don't know how you did it." We did it because cancer is what life handed to us. We had no choice in the matter. But we did find inner reserves we never knew we had and grew stronger for having found them.

Each of us rides the roller coaster of cancer in our own unique way. For all of us, the ride is frightening. But eventually, it slows down and grinds to a halt. We disembark, shaken and weary, and walk away in pursuit of our equilibrium, which, once found, frees us to put the experience of

that horrible ride somewhere in between all the other experiences that make us who we are. But having ridden those
chaotic rails, we are truly summoned to *live*. And that is
exactly what Alex and I are very busy doing!

INFORMATION, SUPPORT AND ADVOCACY

I admit it—I'm partial to the University of Michigan Comprehensive Cancer Center because I got to know the folks there pretty well. But throughout the country, you'll find many fine institutions and dedicated individuals who specialize in treating lymphoma. Some are in private practice. Some work at research institutions where they collaborate with others and work tirelessly to find new treatments with the goal of finding a cure for lymphoma.

There are several sources for information about the disease, but I personally found the most comprehensive to be the Lymphoma Research Foundation (LRF), which is the largest organization devoted to funding lymphoma research and to providing information to patients and families. LRF offers many free educational and support programs and materials to help patients and caregivers understand and cope with the disease. Some of the services include:

- Providing disease-specific information
- Helping to find a clinical trial
- Providing up-to-date information on the latest medical advances

- Matching patients and caregivers with volunteers who have faced a similar type of lymphoma, treatment, or challenge
- Holding conferences and symposiums throughout the country at which some of the country's leading lymphoma experts volunteer their time to teach patients and families about the disease

LRF also works to increase awareness of the disease and to raise funds for research. LRF chapters are growing throughout the country. There are many opportunities to volunteer and to contribute to this organization's important mission.

For more information, visit:
www.lymphoma.org

ACKNOWLEDGEMENTS

Writing a memoir is an intensely personal effort, but it was made infinitely easier by those who read the manuscript and provided feedback and encouragement.

With the greatest of objectivity and compassion, Shannon Sweetnam of Sweetink, Inc., nurtured me through the earliest draft. Written while I was recovering and still under the influence of drugs and doubt, Shannon helped me to eliminate rambling redundancy and irrelevant information. She also encouraged me to include more pertinent details and helped me to structure the story into a piece that resembled a coherent chronology. Most importantly, she left my own words completely intact.

Several friends then read various drafts and encouraged me along the way. In particular, Tom and Marie Fluent, Joe and Lisa Himle, Dr. Arno Kumagai and my daughter Juli deserve special mention for believing in the value of this book. I especially thank Dr. Mark Kaminski and Judy Estes for reading the manuscript for medical accuracy, and for their support of it. Patients and caregivers were my biggest source of inspiration.

Marian Nelson, Joe Aller and Sarah Hart at First Page Publications steadily supported this project and offered sound advice to help me through the publishing process. Sarah was enormously helpful in editing the final draft, and I thank her, too, for leaving my words my own.

As always, my biggest cheerleader was my husband Alex. When I began transforming my journal into a manuscript, he immediately saw that writing gave me a purpose when I had no other, and he encouraged me to continue. At any time, he might have asked me to keep the story to ourselves. He never did. In sickness and in health, he is always there for me with unwavering support, and I thank him for the love and the joy that he brings to my life.

ABOUT THE AUTHOR

Betsy de Parry lives and works with her husband Alex in Ann Arbor, Michigan, where they have a home building company. Both are committed to raising awareness of lymphoma and to helping those who face the disease. Betsy remains in complete remission.

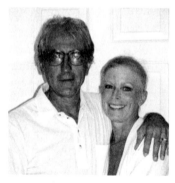

August 2002

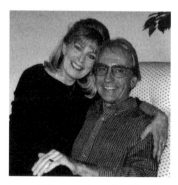

November 2004